FRUITS OF THE WORLD

Dr. Kumar Pati

New Editions Publishing

30982 Huntwood Avenue Suite 208

Hayward, California 94544 USA

dr.kumarpati@bestnutrition.com

The material in this book is intended to disseminate the information to others on fruits and their pictures from various parts of the world. The author, Dr. Abhay Kumar Pati, is a physician who has a degree in Western Medicine as well as in Ayurvedic medicine of India from the J. B. Ray State College & Hospital in Kolkata, India (Kolkata University), one of most prestigious Ayurvedic Colleges in India. Dr. Pati has been living in the U.S. for the past 3 decades and has traveled the world all over. He focuses on prevention and natural therapies than having sickness for treatment and emergency health care. He has a great interest in organic fruits and vegetables as well as food, nutrition as they are the great source of enzyme and nutrients for maintaining a good healthy lifestyle.

Author Pati Abhay Kumar

Edited by: Joanne Dominguez

Design by: Prabin Badhia

Copyright: 2010

Library of Congress Catalog Card Number: 2009911853

ISBN 987-0-615-33458-5

Contents

ACEROLA	9
ACKEE	10
AFRICAN CUCUMBER	11
AMLA, INDIAN GOOSEBERRY	12
APRICOT	13
ASIAN PEARS	14
AUSUBO	15
AVOCADO	16
BAEL FRUIT	17
BANANA	18
BATUAN	19
BILIMBI	20
BLACKBERRY	21
BLACKCURRANT	22
BLUEBERRY	23
BOYSENBERRY	24
BREADFRUIT	25
CALAMANSI	26
CAMACHILE	27
CANISTEL	28
CANTALOUPE	29
CAPEGOOSEBERRY	30
CASHEW FRUIT	31
CEMPEDAK	32
CHERIMOYA	33
CHERRY	34
COCONUT	35

COWBERRY	36
CRANBERRY	37
DALANDAN	38
DATES	39
DRAGON FRUIT	40
DURIAN	41
FEIJOA	42
FIG	43
FUJI APPLE	44
GRANNY SMITH GREEN APPLE	45
GRAPEFRUIT	46
GRAPES	47
GUAPPLE	48
GUAVA	49
HONEYDEW MELON	50
INDIAN JUJUBE	51
JACKFRUIT	52
JAMAICAN CHERRY	53
JAVA PLUM, JAMUN or DUHAT	54
JELLY PALM FRUIT	55
JOCOTE, RED MOMBIN,	56
PURPLE MOMBIN	56
KALUMPIT	57
KIWI FRUIT	58
KUMQUATS	59
LANGSAT, LANZONES	60
LEMON	61
LONGAN	62
LOQUATS	63
LYCHEE	64

MAFAI, BURMESE GRAPE	65
MAMONCILLO	66
MANDARIN ORANGE	67
MANGO	68
MANGOSTEEN	69
MAPRANG	70
MARANG	71
MIRACLE FRUIT	72
NECTARINE	73
NONI	74
ORANGE	75
ORIENTAL MELON	76
OTAHEITE GOOSEBERRY	77
PALMYRA PALM FRUIT	78
PAPAYA	79
PASSION FRUIT	80
PAWPAW	81
PEACH	82
PEARS	83
PEJIBAYE PALM FRUIT	84
PEPINO	85
PERSIMMON	86
PINEAPPLE	87
PLUM	88
POMEGRANATE	89
POMELO	90
PULASAN	91
RAMBUTAN	92
RASPBERRY	93
RED CURRANTS	94

RED DELICIOUS APPLE	95
SALAK	96
SANTOL	97
SAPODILLA, CHICO	98
SEA GRAPE	99
SOURSOP, GUYABANO,	100
GUANABANA	100
STAR APPLE, CAIMITO	101
STARFRUIT, CARAMBOLA	102
STRAWBERRY	103
SUGAR APPLE	104
SURINAM CHERRY	105
SWEET GRANADILLA	106
TAMARILLO	107
TAMARIND	108
TANGERINE	109
TOMATILLOS	110
TOMATO	111
UGLI FRUIT	112
VELVET APPLE, MABOLO	113
WATER LEMON	114
WATERMELON	115
WAX APPLE,	116
WAX JAMBU, MACOPA	116
WHITE CURRANT	117
WOLFBERRY	118

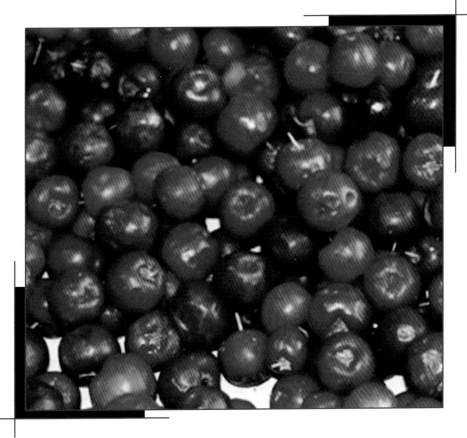

ACEROLA

Acerola (Malpighia glabra) or Acerola is also known as Barbados cherry or wild crapemyrtle, West Indian cherry, Puerto Rican cherry, Antilles cherry, cereza, cerisier and semeruco.

Acerola fruit is a bright red cherry-like fruit containing several small seeds. Mature fruits are soft and pleasant tasting. They contain 80 percent juice. The fruits deteriorate rapidly once removed from the tree. The fruit is edible and widely consumed in the species' native area, and is cultivated elsewhere for its high vitamin C content.

Acerola has now been successfully introduced in sub-tropical areas throughout the world (Southeast Asia, India, South America), and some of the largest plantings are in Brazil.

Therapeutic use: This fruit is low in saturated fat and sodium, and very low in cholesterol. It is also a good source of dietary fiber, riboflavin, folate, magnesium, potassium and copper, and a very good source of vitamin A and vitamin C.

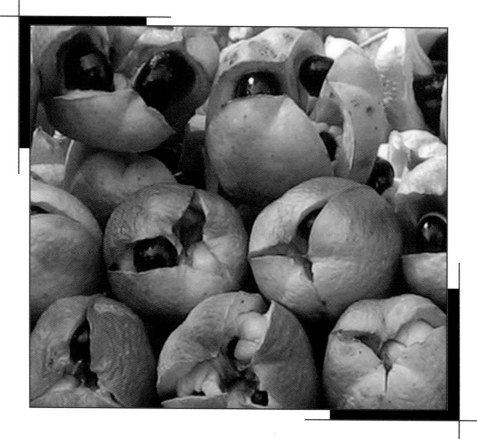

ACKEE

Ackee or Akee (Blighia sapida) is a tropical fruit belonging to the Sapindaceae family. It has its origin in West Africa but has traversed the Atlantic Ocean making the Caribbean its home.

It is a pear-shaped fruit that when ripens, turns from green to a bright red to yellow-orange, and splits open to reveal three large, shiny black seeds, surrounded by soft, creamy or spongy, white to yellow flesh – arili. The fruit typically weighs 100-200 grams.

The fruit of the ackee is not edible in its entirety. Only the inner, fleshy yellow arils are consumed. The shiny black seeds at the tips of the arils, and the bright red pod enclosing 3 or 4 arils are discarded. Ackee pods should be allowed to ripen and open naturally on the tree before picking. Prior to cooking, the ackee arils must be cleaned, washed, boiled and the water discarded: raw ackees and the inner red tissue of the ripe ackee arils contain potent alkaloid toxins (Hypoglycins A and B) which can produce a syndrome of vomiting, seizures, and fatal hypoglycemia known as Jamaican vomiting sickness.

Therapeutic use: Though it may be poisonous when improperly prepared, ackee has high nutritional value and is rich in essential fatty acids, vitamin A, zinc and protein.

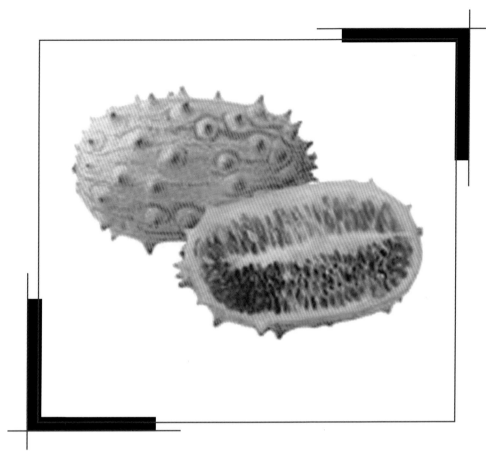

AFRICAN CUCUMBER

African Cucumber (Cucumis metuliferus), also known as kiwano, jelly melon, horned melon or melano, is a fruit that can be best described as melon with horns. It originated in the Kalahari Desert and is now present in California and New Zealand.

The spiny fruit which turns bright orange when it is ripe, has a subtle citrus or banana-like flavor that the fruit pulp, a lime green jelly-like flesh can be strained to make a juice. The fruit makes an excellent garnish and its long keeping qualities make it suitable for decorative purposes.

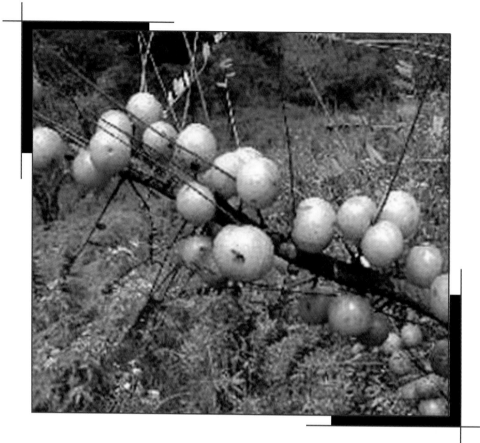

AMLA, INDIAN GOOSEBERRY

Amla (Phyllantus emblica) is also usually called Indian gooseberry. Other names include heikru in Manipuri, nelli in Sinhala, nellikka in Malayalam, amlakhi in Assamese, usirikai in Telugu and nellikaai in Tamil and Kannada as well as aonla, aola, ammalaki, dharty, aamvala, aawallaa, emblic, emblic myrobalan, Malacca tree, nillika, and nellikya in various other languages.

The fruit is nearly spherical, light greenish yellow, quite smooth and hard in appearance, with 6 vertical stripes or furrows. The taste of Indian gooseberry is sour, bitter and astringent, and is quite fibrous. In India, it is common to eat gooseberries steeped in salt water and turmeric to make the sour fruits palatable.

Therapeutic use: Amla is a natural, efficacious, antioxidant with the richest natural source of Vitamin C. The fruit contains the highest amount of Vitamin C in natural form and cytokine like substances identified as zeatin, z. riboside, z. nucleotide. Its fruit is acrid, cooling, refrigerant, diuretic and laxative. The dried fruit is useful in hemorrhage, diarrhea and dysentery.It is antibacterial and its astringent properties prevent infection and help in the healing of ulcers. It is used as a laxative to relieve constipation in piles. It is used in the treatment of leukorrhea and artherosclerosis.

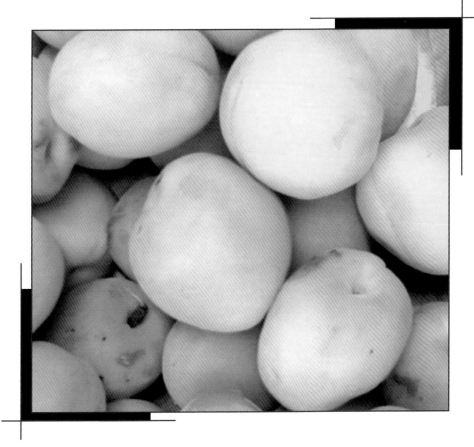

APRICOT

Apricot (Prunus armeniaca), a species of Prunus classified with the plum, is a small, sweet fruit with a golden orange color. A ripe apricot can be recognized by its fairly firm skin, and it will be plump and juicy when it is at its best. A drupe, about 1.5"-2.5" wide, with a prominent suture, having light pubescent or a nearly glabrous surface. The pit is generally smooth, enclosing a single seed. Flesh color is mostly orange, but a few white-fleshed cultivars exist.

Apricots have an extremely short shelf-life of only 1-2 weeks at 0 degrees C and 90% relative humidity. Most of the US crop is not sold fresh; drying and canning are popular options for apricots since they are so perishable.

Therapeutic use: Apricot is an excellent source of Vitamins A (beta-carotene) and C. Apricots are also a good source of iron, potassium, phosphorus and calcium.

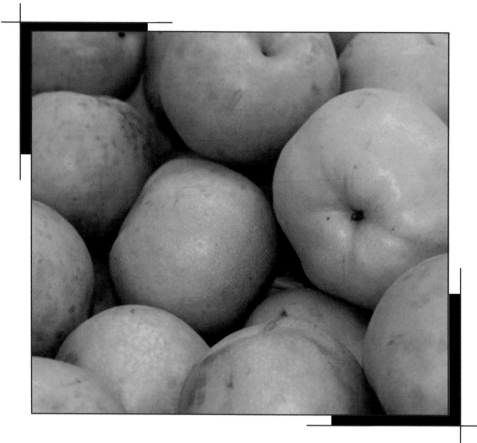

ASIAN PEARS

Asian pears (Pyrus pyrifolia), sometimes referred to as "apple pears", are species native to China, Japan and Korea. Other names that this fruit goes by are Chinese pear, Japanese pear, Sand, Nashi, African pear, Korean pear, Taiwan pear, bapple, papple bae, and li (China). In South Asia, the fruit is known as nashipati or nashpati. It is cultivated throughout East Asia, as well as in Australia, India, New Zealand and other countries.

Asian pears differ from the traditional European ones. These pears are usually round, firm to touch when ripe, and are ready to eat after harvest. These pears will be crisp, juicy, and slightly sweet with some tartness, especially near the core. They are commonly served raw.

There are 3 types of Asian pears. They are 1) round or flat fruit with green-to-yellow skin, 2) round or flat fruit with bronze-colored skin and a light bronze-russet, 3) pear-shaped fruit with green or russet skin.

Therapeutics use: Pears contain about 16 percent carbohydrate and negligible amounts of fat and protein. They are good sources of the B-complex vitamins and also contain vitamin C in addition, they contain small amounts of phosphorus and iodine.

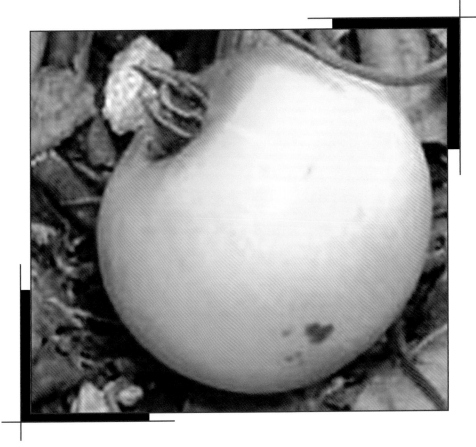

AUSUBO

Ausubo (Manilkara bidentata), also known as balata, is a medium sized, yellow skinned fruit, about two inches across, bearing many similarities to the sapodilla.

Ausubo fruits can be eaten fresh.

It is native to Puerto Rico, widely distribute throughout the West Indies, and ranges from Mexico through Panama to northern South America, including the Guianas and Venezuela, to Peru, and to northern Brazil.

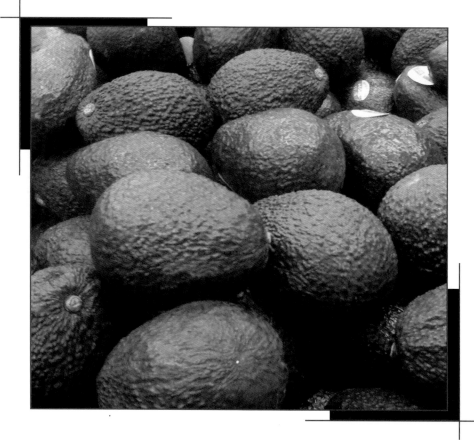

AVOCADO

Avocado (Persea Americana), also known as palta or aguacate (Spanish), butter pear or alligator pear, is a tree native to the Caribbean, Mexico, South America and Central America.

The fruit ranges from more or less round to egg or pear shaped, typically the size of a temperate-zone pear or larger, on the outside bright green to green-brown (or almost black) in color. The flesh is typically greenish yellow to golden yellow when ripe. It is not sweet, but fatty, distinctly yet subtly flavored and of smooth, almost creamy texture.

Avocado is almost always served raw, especially in Mexican dishes such as guacamole.

Therapeutic use: Naturally sodium-free and cholesterol free, avocados act as a nutrient booster by enabling the body to absorb more fat-soluble nutrients, such as alpha and beta-carotene as well as lutein, in foods that are eaten with the fruit.

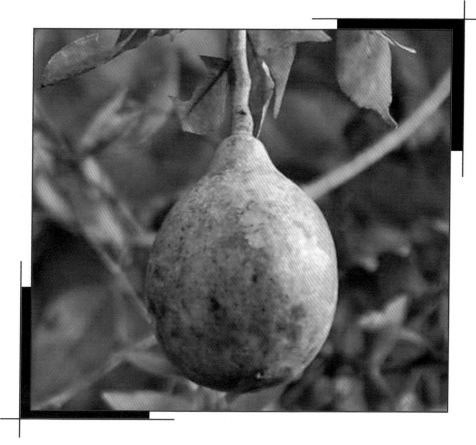

BAEL FRUIT

Bael Fruit (Aegle marmelos Correa), though more prized for it`s medicinal virtues than it`s edible quality is, nevertheless, of sufficient importance as an edible fruit. It is also called Bengal quince, Indian quince, golden apple, holy fruit, stone apple, bel, bela, sirphal, maredoo and other dialectal names in India; matum and mapin in Thailand; phneou or pnoi in Cambodia; bau nau in Vietnam; bilak or maj pahit in Malaya; modjo in Java; orange du Malabar in French; marmelos in Potuguese. Sometimes it is also called elephant apple.

Bael fruit is round and roughly the size of a baseball. The fruit starts out gray-green and turns a pale yellow when it matures. When split open, the fruit will reveal pale orange pulp separated by thick, dark orange walls. The fruit is also studded with resinous hairy seeds, enclosed in an envelope of mucilage. The odor of the fruit can be off putting to some.

This fruit can be eaten raw or cooked, and is often utilized in an unripe stage.

Therapeutic use: When unripe, the fruit can be used to treat diarrhea, while the ripened fruit is a laxative. An effusion of bael is regarded as an effective food remedy for peptic ulcers.

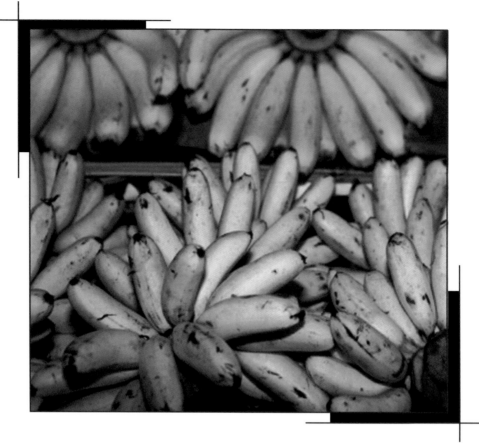

BANANA

Banana is the common name for a type of fruit and also the herbaceous plants of the genus Musa which produce this commonly eaten fruit. They are native to the tropical region of Southeast Asia.

Bananas come in a variety of sizes and colors when ripe, including yellow, purple and red. Bananas can be eaten raw though some varieties are generally cooked first. Depending on cultivar and ripeness, the flesh can vary in taste from starchy to sweet, and texture from firm to mushy. Unripe or green bananas and plaintains are used for cooking various dishes.

Therapeutic use: Banana is a very good source of dietary fiber, Vitamin C, Potassium and Manganese, and a very good source of Vitamin B6.

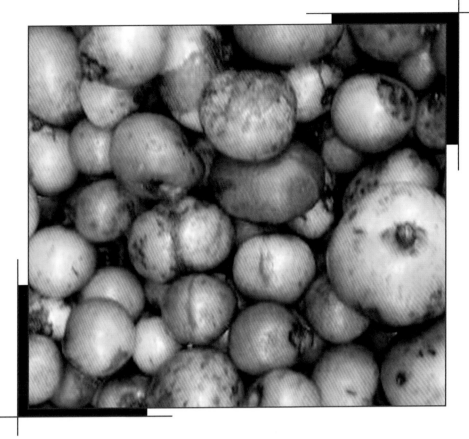

BATUAN

Batuan (Garcinia binucao) is a fruit that is greenish, yellowish, somewhat rounded, and 4 centimeters or more in diameter. They have a firm outer covering and contain a very acid pulp and several seeds.

This fruit is usually used as a souring agent to dishes.

Other local names include ballok (Benguet); balukut (Ilocos Norte); bangkok (Zambales); batuan (Negros, Guimaras & Burias island); bilukao (Rizal, Bataan, Batangas, Camarines); binukao (Laguna, Bataan); buragris (Camarines); kamang-si (Tayabas); haras (Capiz); kandis (Palawan); kanumai, kulilem (Cagayan); maninila (Albay).

This species is common and widely distributed throughout Luzon and the Visayan islands of the Philippines.

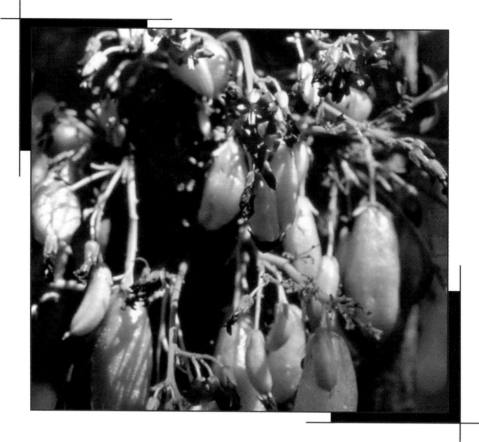

BILIMBI

Bilimbi (Averrhoa bilimbi), is closely allied to the carambola but quite different in appearance, manner of fruiting, flavor and uses. Bilimbi is the common name in India; belimbing asam, belimbing buloh, b'ling or billing billing in Malaya, belimbing besu, balimbing, blimbing or blimbing wuluh in Indonesia; taling pling or kaling pring in Thailand. In Haiti, it is called blimbin; in Jamaica, bumbling plum; in Cuba, it is grosella china; in El Salvador and Nicaragua, mimbro; in Costa Rica, mimbro or tirguro; in Venezuela, vinagrillo; in Surinam and Guyana, birambi; in Argentina, pepino de Indias; in French, carambolier bilimbi or cornichon des Indes and in Philippines, it is called kamias or iba.

Multi-lobed, oblong fruit with a pale green waxy skin and crunchy but watery flesh, very similar to the star fruit, although the flesh is much more acidic.

The most common use for the fruits is a flavoring for prepared fish and meat dishes. Fruits are also used for beverages and preserves. They are quite acidic and unlike the star fruit, are usually not eaten fresh out of hand.

Native to Indonesia. Grows semi-wild throughout southeast Asia. The tree is also cultivated in parts of southeast Asia.

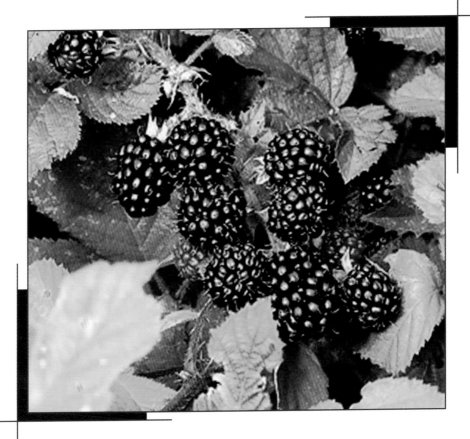

BLACKBERRY

Blackberry is an aggregate fruit from a bramble bush, genus Rubus in the rose family Rosaceae. It is widespread, and well known group of several hundred species, many of which are closely related apomictic microspecies native throughout the temperate Northern hemisphere.

Ripe blackberry fruit is usually black or dark purple, and often sweet and flavorful.

Therapeutic use: Blackberries rank highly among fruits for antioxidant strength, particularly due to their dense contents of polyphenolic compounds, such as ellagic acid, tannins, ellagitannins, quercetin, gallic acid, anthocyanins and cyanidins.

Blackberries are notable for their high nutritional contents of dietary fiber, vitamin C, vitamin K, folic acid – B vitamin, and the essential mineral, manganese.

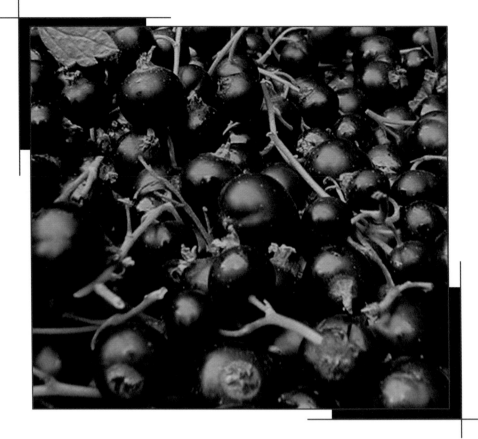

BLACKCURRANT

Blackcurrant (Ribes nigrum) is a species of Ribes berry native to central and northern Europe and northern Asia. It is also known as French "cassis".

The fruit is an edible berry 1cm diameter, very dark purple in color, almost black, with a glossy skin and persistent calyx at the apex, and contains several seeds dense in nutrients.

Blackcurrant berries have a distinctive sweet and sharp taste popular in jam, juice, ice cream, and liquour. Other than being juiced and used in jellies, syrups, and cordials, blackcurrants are used in cooking because their astringent nature brings out flavor in many sauces, meat dishes and desserts.

Therapeutic use: The fruit has an extraordinarily high vitamin C content (302% of the Daily Value per 100g, table), good levels of potassium, phosphorus, iron and vitamin B5, and a broad range of other essential nutrients.

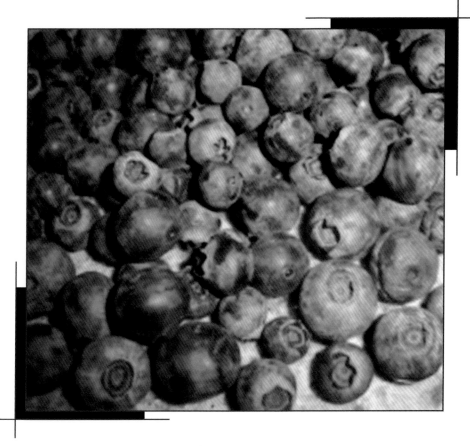

BLUEBERRY

Blueberries are flowering plants of the genus Vaccinium with dark-blue, purple or black berries. Species in the section Cyanococcus are the most common fruits sold as "blueberries" and are mainly native to North America.

The fruit is a false berry 5-16mm diameter with flared crown at the end; they are pale greenish at first, then reddish-purple, and finally blue on ripening. They have a sweet taste when mature, with variable acidity.

Blueberries are sold fresh or processed as individually quick frozen fruit, puree, juice, or dried or infused berries which in turn may be used in a variety of consumer goods such as jellies, jams, pies, muffins, snack foods, and cereals.

Therapeutic use: This fruit is a very good source of Vitamin C, Vitamin K and Manganese.

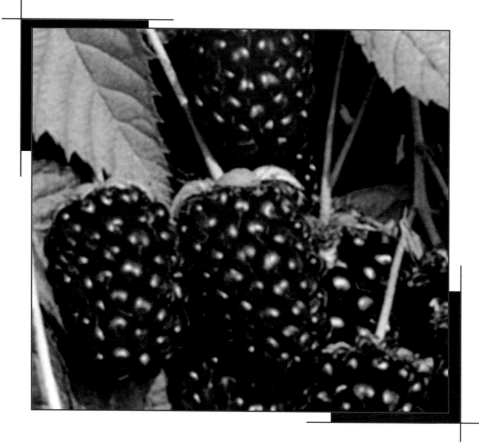

BOYSENBERRY

Boysenberry (Rubus ursinus x idaeus) is the common name for a hybrid plant of the blackberry/ raspberry genus Rubus and characterized by a relatively large fruit, with large seeds and a deep maroon or reddish-black color. The boysenberry is a human creation achieved through a selective crossing by a horticulturist Rudolph Boysen in the early 1920s.

Boysenberries has a rich, sweet and tart flavor. This unique berry may be eaten fresh, used in jams, preserves, pies and syrups or even made into a wine.

Therapeutic use: This fruit is also nutritious being rich in vitamin C, fiber, calcium and anthocyanins (which work as antioxidants), and a source of iron.

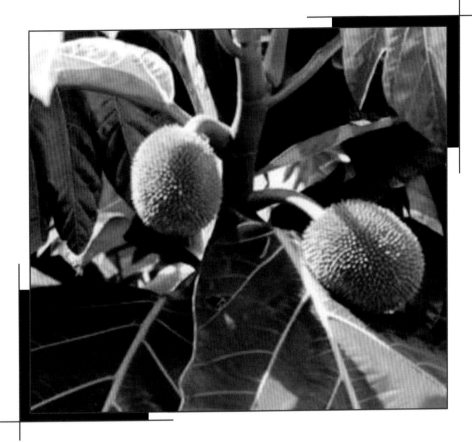

BREADFRUIT

Breadfruit (Artocarpus altilis), native to the Malay peninsula and western Pacific island, is large (8 to 10 inches in diameter), has bumpy green skin and rather bland-tasting, cream-colored center. The breadfruit is closely related to the breadnut and the jackfruit. It is called Kada Chakka or Cheema (Sheema) Chakka in the Malayalam language and Jeegujje/Geegujje/Jigujje in Tulu.

It is picked and eaten before it ripens and becomes too sweet. Like squash, breadfruit can be baked, grilled, fried or boiled and served as a sweet or savory dish. It can also be ground up and made into bread.

Therapeutic use: A 200g portion is a rich source of Vitamin C; a source of iron and Vitamin B and supplies 220kcal (925kJ).

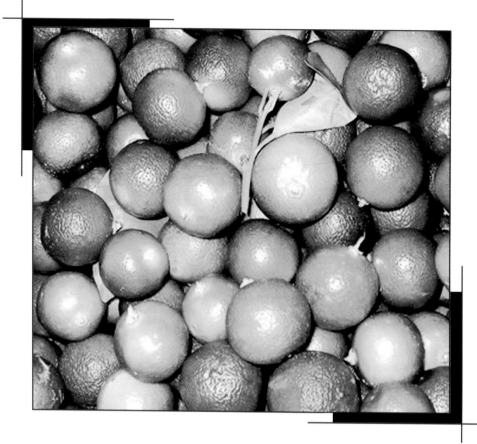

CALAMANSI

Calamansi or Calamondin (citrofortunella microcarpa) belongs to the citrus family. It is a fruit tree native in the Philippines.

The fruit is usually small and round. The rind may be thin or thick. It`s juice is used as a flavoring ingredient or as an additive in various food preparations. The pulp can be utilized in beverages, syrups, concentrates and purees.

Therapeutic use: It is a rich source of Vitamin C. With its alkalinizing effect, calamansi helps blood circulate energy and facilitates normal digestion.

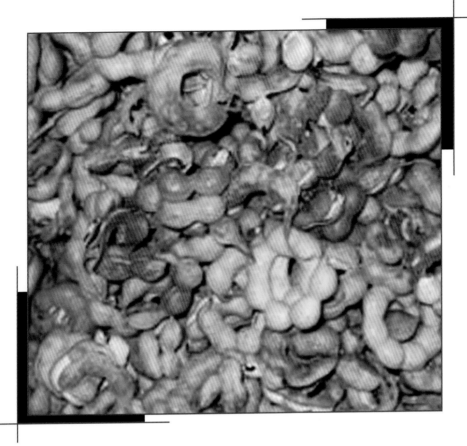

CAMACHILE

Camachile (Pithecellobium dulce), is a common thorny tropical American tree that originated from Mexico and other Central and South American countries where it is known as Guamachil. It is also called Manila Tamarind in English, opiuma in Hawaii, kamatsile in Philippines and Jungle jalebi and Madras thorn. Also called blackbead, sweet inga, sweet tamarind.

The flowers are greenish-white, fragrant, sessile and reach about 12cm long though looks shorter due to coiling. The flowers produce a pod with an edible pulp. The seeds are black.

The camachile fruit or pods contain a white acidic and sweetish pulp that is eaten raw or prepared as a beverage.

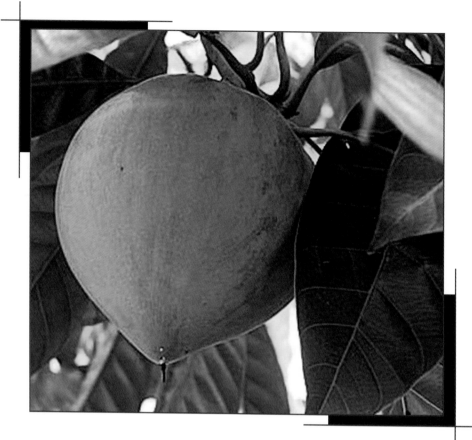

CANISTEL

Canistel (Pouteria campechiana), is also called egg fruit, yellow sapote (Cuba, Hawaii, Jamaica, Puerto Rico, Bahamas, Florida); canistel, siguapa, zapotillo (Costa Rica); costiczapotl, custiczapotl fruta de huevo, zapote amarillo (Colombia); cakixo, canizte, kanis, kaniste, hantzé, kantez, limoncillo, mamee ciruela, zapotillo de montana (Guatemala); huevo vegetal (Puerto Rico, Venezuela); mammee sapota, eggfruit, ti-es (Bahamas); mamey cerera, mamey cerilla, mamee ciruela, kanizte (Belize); atzapotl (the fruit), atzapolquahuitl (the tree), caca de niño, cozticzapotl, cucumu, mamey de Campechi, mamey de Cartagena, huicumo, huicon, kan 'iste', kanixte, kanizte, palo huicon, zapote amarillo, zapote de niño, zapote borracho (drunken sapote, perhaps because the fallen fruits ferment on the ground); zapote mante, zubul (Mexico); guaicume, guicume, zapotillo, zapotillo amarillo (El Salvador); zapote amarillo (Nicaragua); boracho, canistel, chesa (Philippines).

The exterior of a canistel fruit is a glossy skin that, upon ripening, varies in yellow and orange tones. Canistel fruit is soft, rather than crisp, and it is not particularly juicy. Inside of the fruit are a few large glossy black or dark brown seeds.

The flesh of canistel fruits are sometimes incorporated into desserts, such as ice creams and puddings. The fruit is also enjoyed when tossed with mayonnaise, salt, pepper, and a citrus juice such as lemon or lime.

Therapeutic use: Like most fruits, canistel fruits are rich in a number of vitamins and nutrients. They are particularly rich in carotene and niacin. They also have a good amount of ascorbic acid.

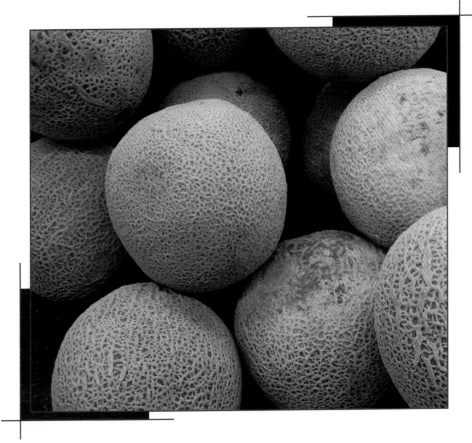

CANTALOUPE

Cantaloupe (Cucumis melo), also called muskmelon or rockmelon, is characterized by a webbed surface. Cantaloupes have a smooth and lumpy skin with deep ridges.

Because the surface of a cantaloupe can contain harmful bacteria - in particular, salmonella – it is always a good idea to wash melon throughly before cutting and consumption. The rind is rich in nutrients so the whole melon may be juiced.

Therapeutic use: This fruit has significant amounts of Vitamin A and C, are good source of potassium and contain small amounts of many other minerals. Cantaloupes are a source of polyphenol antioxidants, chemicals which are known to provide certain health benefits to the cardiovascular system and immune system.

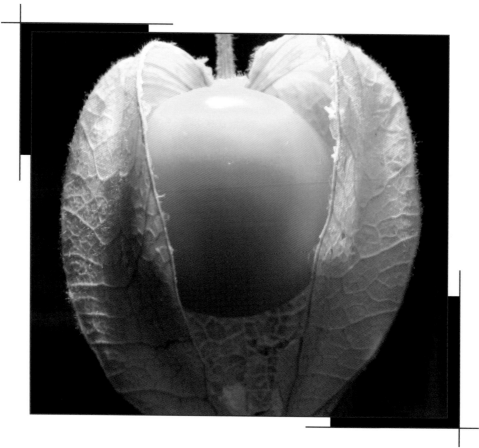

CAPEGOOSEBERRY

Cape gooseberry (Physalis peruviana), also called goldenberry, husk cherry, Peruvian ground cherry, poha, poha berry, is native to Brazil but long ago became naturalized in the highlands of Peru and Chile.

After the flower falls, the calyx expands, forming a straw-colored husk much larger than the fruit enclosed, which take 70 to 80 days to mature. The fruit is a berry with smooth, waxy, orange-yellow skin and juicy pulp containing numerous very small yellowish seeds. As the fruits ripen, they begin to drop to the ground, but will continue to mature and change from green to the golden-yellow of the mature fruit. The unripe fruit is said to be poisonous to some people. The fruit is harvested when it falls to the ground, but not all fallen fruits may be in the same stage of maturity and must be held until they ripen.

The ripe fruit can be eaten out of hand or used in a number of other ways. The unique flavor of the fresh fruit makes it an interesting ingredient in salads and cooked dishes. Cape gooseberries cooked with apples or ginger make a very distinctive dessert. The fruits are also an attractive sweet when dipped in chocolate or other glazes or pricked and rolled in sugar. The high pectin content makes cape gooseberry a good preserve and jam product that can be used as a dessert topping. The fruit also dries into tasty "raisins".

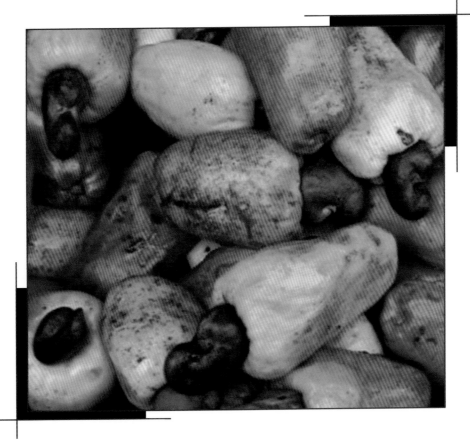

CASHEW FRUIT

Cashew fruit (Anacardium occidentale), is also called maranon in most Spanish speaking countries, but merey in Venezuela; caju or cajueiro in Portuguese, kaju in Hindi and kasuy in Philippines.

The fragrant, reddish flowers grow in clusters, and the pear shaped fruits, called cashew apples, are reddish or yellowish. At the end of each fruit is a kidney shaped ovary, the nut, with a hard double shell.

Cashew apples are sometimes made locally into drinks, wines and pickles. In some countries they are also osmo-sol dried to produce a date-like caramel.

While the tree is native to central and South America, it is now widely distributed throughout the tropics, particularly in many parts of Africa and Asia.

Therapeutic use: This fruit is very low in cholesterol and sodium. It is a good source of Magnesium, Phosphorus, Copper and Manganese.

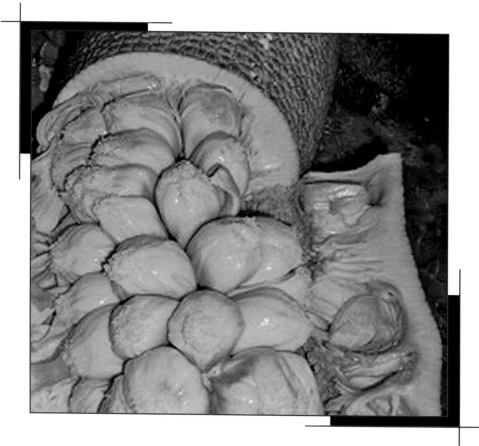

CEMPEDAK

Cempedak or Chempedak (Artocarpus integer) is a species of tree and its fruit in the family Moraceae. It is native to Southeast Asia, occurring from West Malaysia east to West Irian on the island of New Guinea. It has been introduced to Queensland.

The sausage-shaped fruit range from 22 to 50 centimeters in length and 10 to 17 cm across. The edible arils surrounding the large seeds are yellow, orange or green in color. The taste of the fruit is similar to the related jackfruit and breadfruit with a hint of durian. The sweet, juicy pulp surrounds the seeds in a thick layer between the husk and an inedible core. The green skin is thin and leathery, patterned with hexagons that are either flat or raised protuberances like jackfruit skin.

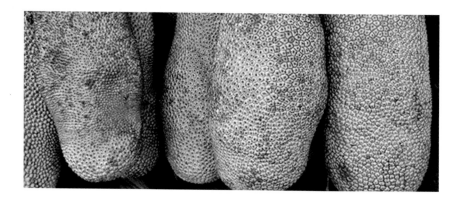

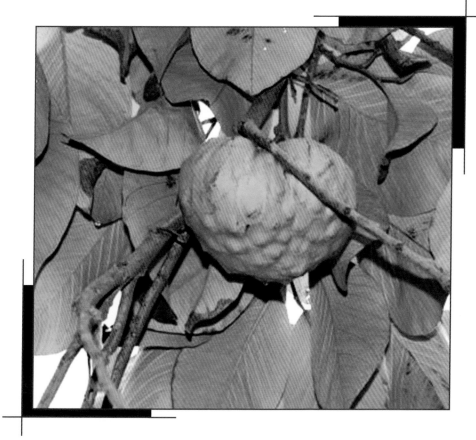

CHERIMOYA

Cherimoya (Annona cherimola) is a species of Annona native to the Andean-highland valleys of Ecuador and Peru. Other names of cherimoya are mang cau in Vietnam, nona in Malay, srikaya in Indonesia, laxmanphal in Hindi, kachiman in Haitian Creole,

The fruit is oval, often slightly oblique, 10-20 cm long and 7-10 cm diameter, with a smooth or slightly tuberculated skin. The fruit is fleshy and soft, sweet, white in color, with a sherbet-like texture, which gives it its secondary name, custard apple. Some characterize the flavor as a blend of banana, pineapple, and strawberry. Others describe it as tasting like commercial bubblegum. Similar in size to a grapefruit, it has large, glossy, dark seeds that are easily removed. The seeds are poisonous if crushed open and can be used as an insecticide.

The flesh of the ripe cherimoya is most commonly eaten out of-hand or scooped with a spoon from the cut open fruit.

Therapeutic use: This fruit is very low in cholesterol and sodium. It is a good source of dietary fiber, Vitamin B6 and Potassium, and a very good source of Vitamin C.

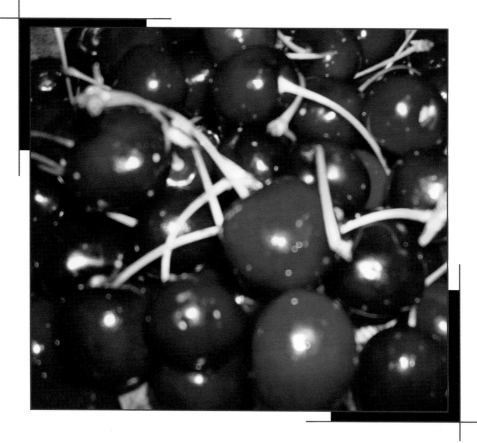

CHERRY

Cherry is a fleshy fruit (drupe) that contains a single stony seed. The cherry belongs to the family Rosaceae, genus Prunus, along with almonds, peaches plums, apricots and bird cherries.

The United States is the world's biggest producer, consumer and exporter of cherries.

Therapeutic use: Cherries are a good source of Vitamins A and C and potassium, and sour cherries contain more Beta carotene than the sweet. They also contain pectin and anthocyanins, which are flavonoids linked to the prevention of cancer and heart diseases.

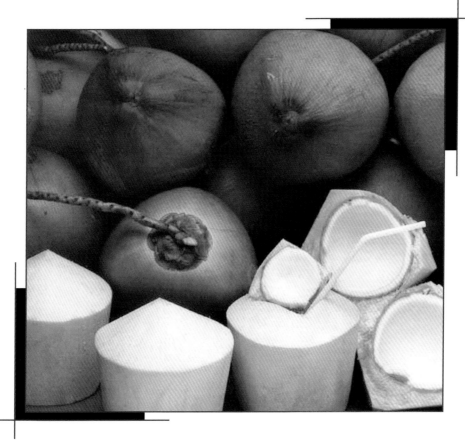

COCONUT

Coconut (Cocos nucifera) is the fruit of the coconut palm. The fruit-bearing palms are native to Malaysia, Polynesia and southern Asia, and are now also prolific in South America, India, the Pacific Islands, Hawaii and Florida.

The egg-shaped (ovoid) fruits are up to 35 cm long and 30 cm wide. They have a green color which turns to brown in mature fruits. The outer part of the fruit is a thick fibrous husk. Inside this is the almost spherical nut which has a hard woody shell that is rather hairy on the outside. The nut can measure from 12 to 20 cm in diameter and up to 25 cm long. On one end of the nut are three round soft spots which are called the eyes. Inside the nut is a layer of white flesh, which is called copra. This layer of meat is very thin in younger fruits, and becomes harder and thicker (up to 2 cm) in older fruits. The central space of the nut is filled with a sweet liquid, which is called coconut milk. Especially the younger fruits contain a lot of this coconut water.

The coconut fruit has many food uses for its water, milk, meat, sugar, and oil. It also functions as its own dish and cup.

Therapeutic use: This fruit is very low in cholesterol and sodium. It is also a very good source of Manganese.

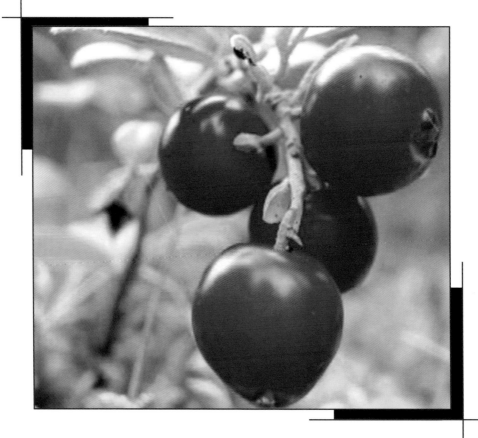

COWBERRY

Cowberry (Vaccinium vitis-idaea) often called lingonberry, foxberry, mountain cranberry, mountain bilberry, partridgeberry and redberry.

It is seldom cultivated, but the fruits are commonly collected in the wild. The native habitat is the circumboreal forests of northern Eurasia and North America, extending from temperate into subarctic climates.

The berries are quite tart, so they are almost always cooked and sweetened before eating in the form of lingonberry jam, compote, juice, or syrup. The raw fruits are also frequently simply mashed with sugar, which preserves most of their nutrients and flavor and even enables storing them at room temperature (in closed but not necessarily sealed containers).

Theraputic use: Cowberries contain plentiful organic acids, vitamin C, provitamin A (as beta carotene), B vitamins (B1, B2, B3), and the elements potassium, calcium, magnesium, and phosphorus. In addition to these healthful nutrients, Lingonberries also contain phytochemicals that are thought to counteract urinary-tract infections, and the seeds are rich in Omega-3 fatty acids.

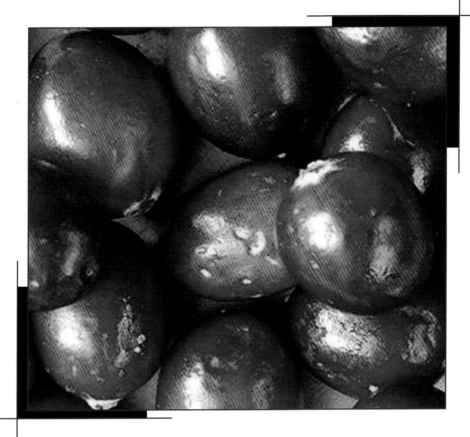

CRANBERRY

Cranberry (Vaccinium macrocarpon Ait) is a native American fruit. Its native range extends in temperate climate zones from the East Coast to the Central U. S. and Canada and from Southern Canada in the north to the Appalachians in the south. Another name used in northeastern Canada is mossberry.

Fresh cranberries can be frozen at home, and will keep up to nine months; they can be used directly in recipes without thawing. Usually, cranberries as fruit are served as a compote or jelly, often known generically as cranberry sauce. Cranberry juice is a major use of cranberries; it is usually either sweetened to reduce its natural severe tartness and make "cranberry juice cocktail" or blended with other fruit juices.

Therapeutic use: Cranberries have moderate levels of vitamin C, dietary fiber and the essential dietary mineral, manganese, as well as a balanced profile of other essential micronutrients. It is a source of polyphenol antioxidants, phytochemicals under active research for possible benefits to the cardiovascular system, immune system and as anti-cancer agents.

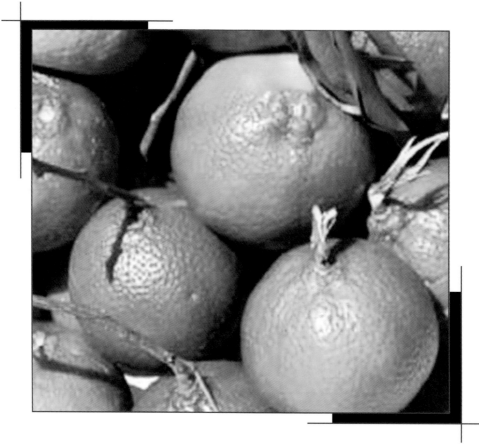

DALANDAN

Dalandan (Citrus aurantium), or Philippine orange, is a type of citrus fruit. This fruit has been a product of the Bicol, Quezon and Mindoro regions.

The fruit is usually medium-sized and spherical to slightly obovate. It tastes like mandarin with a sweeter taste profile and juicier than orange.

Therapeutic use: It is a good source of Vitamin C and rich in flavonoids.

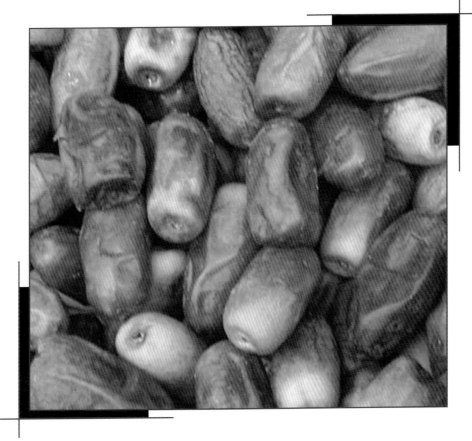

DATES

Dates (Phoenix dactylifera) is a fruit from the date palm with an oval-cylindrical shape, 3-7 cm long and 2-3 cm diameter, and when unripe, range from bright red to bright yellow in color, depending on variety.

They are crispy, sweet and slightly pungent. Most tree-ripened dates are dried before they are sent to markets.

The date palm is native to desert regions of Northern Africa and the Middle East, although it is also cultivated in other parts of the world. This is truly a palm of desert oasis.

Therapeutic use: It is rich in natural fibers, and also comprise a lot of other nutrients, like oil, calcium, sulfur, iron, potassium, phosphorous, manganese, copper, magnesium, etc.

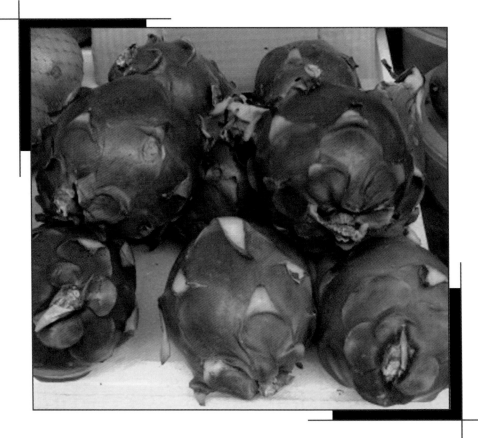

DRAGON FRUIT

Dragon fruit (Stenocereus queretaroensis) is a beautiful fruit grown in Southeast Asia, Mexico, Central and South America, and Israel. Also known as pitaya or pitahaya, it is actually the fruit of a type of cactus.

The fruit comes in 3 colors: 2 have pink skin, but with different colored flesh (one white, the other red), while another type is yellow with white flesh.

Dragon fruit tastes wonderful, sweet and crunchy, with a flavor that's like a cross between kiwi and pear. To prepare a pitaya for consumption, cut the fruit vertically into two halves. From here, either cut the halves into watermelon-like slices, or scoop out the two white fleshy halves with a tablespoon.

Therapeutic use: Dragon fruit is low in calories and offers numerous nutrients, including Vitamin C, phosphorus, calcium, plus fiber and antioxidants.

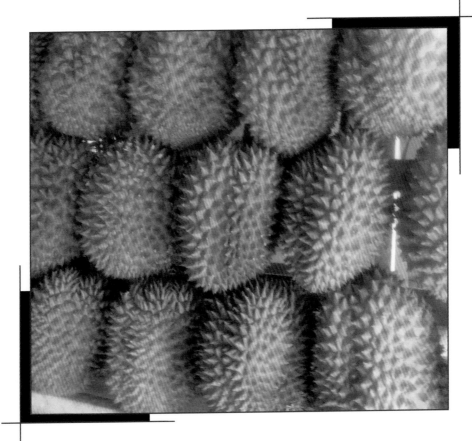

DURIAN

Durian (Durio zibethinus), is a large, spiky fruit, native to the tropical rainforests of Southeast Asia where it is known as "the king of the fruits".

The durian is distinctive for it`s large size, unique odour and formidable thorn-covered husk. The fruit can grow as large as 30cm (12 in) long and 15cm (6 in) diameter, and it typically weighs one to three kilograms (2 to 7 lbs). It`s shape ranges from oblong to round, the color of it's husk green to brown, and it's flesh pale-yellow to red, depending on the species.

Besides eating durian raw, some people use it to make soup, candy, pastries and ice cream. They also eat the seed, usually sliced and fried in oil.

Therapeutic use: Durian is a nutritious food packed with minerals, proteins, and fats.

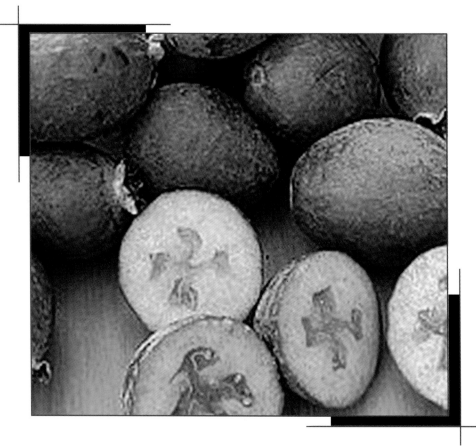

FEIJOA

Feijoa (Feijoa sellowiana), also known as pineapple guava or guavasteen, is a green colored fruit, ellipsoid and about the size of a chicken's egg. It has a sweet, aromatic flavor. The flesh is juicy and is divided into a clear jelly-like seed pulp and a firmer, slightly gritty, opaque flesh nearer the skin. Feijoa fruit has a distinctive smell.

The fruit is usually eaten by cutting it in half, then scooping out the pulp with a spoon or can be torn or bitten in half, and the contents squeezed out and consumed.

This fruit has originated from the highlands of Southern Brazil and parts of Colombia, Uruguay and northern Argentina. It is widely cultivated as a garden plant and fruiting tree in New Zealand, and can be found as a garden plant in Australia and Azerbaijan.

Therapeutic use: This food is very low in cholesterol and sodium. It is also a good source of Folate, and a very good source of Vitamin C.

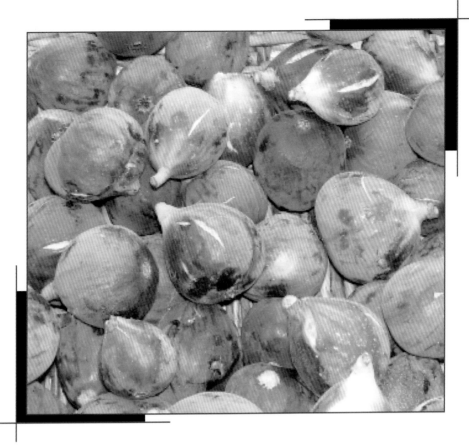

FIG

Fig (Ficus carica), is believed to be indigenous to Western Asia and to have been distributed by man throughout the Mediterranean area.

The matured "fruit" has a tough peel (pure green, green suffused with brown, brown or purple), often cracking upon ripeness, and exposing the pulp beneath. The interior is a white inner rind containing a seed mass bound with jelly-like flesh. The edible seeds are numerous and generally hollow, unless pollinated. Pollinated seeds provide the characteristic nutty taste of dried figs.

Figs can be eaten fresh or dried, and used in jam-making. Most commercial production is in dried or otherwise processed forms, since the ripe fruit does not transport well, and once picked does not keep well.

Therapeutic use: Figs are one of the highest plant sources of calcium and fiber. According to USDA data for the Mission variety, dried figs are richest in fiber, copper, manganese, magnesium, potassium, calcium, and vitamin K, relative to human needs. They have smaller amounts of many other nutrients. Figs have a laxative effect and contain many antioxidants. They are good source of flavonoids and polyphenols.

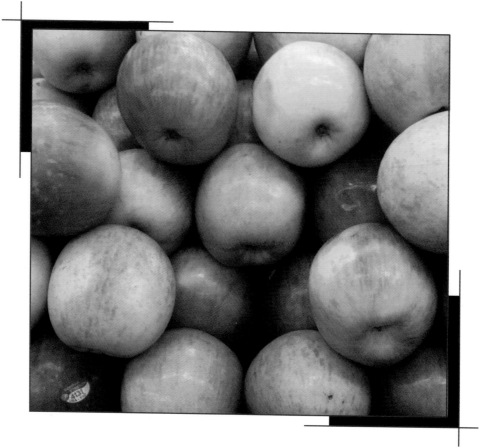

FUJI APPLE

Fuji apple is an apple cultivar which is a cross between two American apple varieties, the Red Delicious and Ralls Janet bred at a Japanese research station.

Fuji contains between 15 to 18 percent sugar and has a dense flesh, making it sweeter and crispier than many other apple varieties. Fuji also has a very long shelf life compared to other apples even without refrigeration.

It is excellent for fresh eating, very good for salads, pies, baking and freezing.

Therapeutic use: Fuji apples have a high amount of flavonoids, in particular one called quercitin. This greatly reduces the risk of heart attack and heart disease, by as much as 20 percent according to a recent study in Finland. It also contains Vitamin C, helps greatly reduce cholesterol levels which protects the heart and arteries. Apples get their sweet taste from a natural sugar known as fructose. Along with the fiber in a fuji apple, the fructose breaks down slowly, which helps to maintain a low blood sugar level.

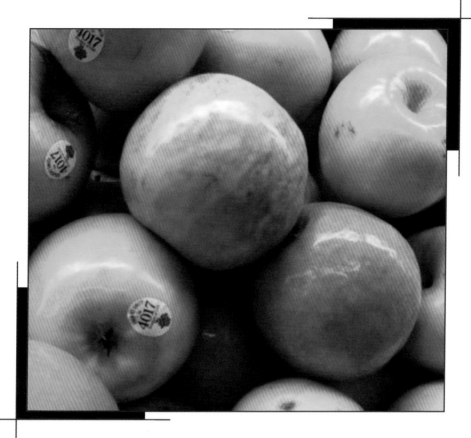

GRANNY SMITH GREEN APPLE

Granny Smith Green Apple is a tip-bearing apple cultivar. It originated in Australia in 1868 from a chance seedling propagated by Maria Ann Smith, where the name "Granny Smith" comes from.

Granny Smith apples are light green in color. They are crisp, juicy, tart apples which are excellent for both cooking and eating raw. They are also flavored for salads because the slices do not brown as quickly as other varieties. It also tends to have a harder texture than other green apples.

Widely propagated in New Zealand, it was introduced to the United Kingdom circa in 1935 and the United States in 1972 by Grady Auvil.

Therapeutics use: Apples are very low in Saturated Fat, Cholesterol and Sodium. They're also a good source of Dietary Fiber and Vitamin C.

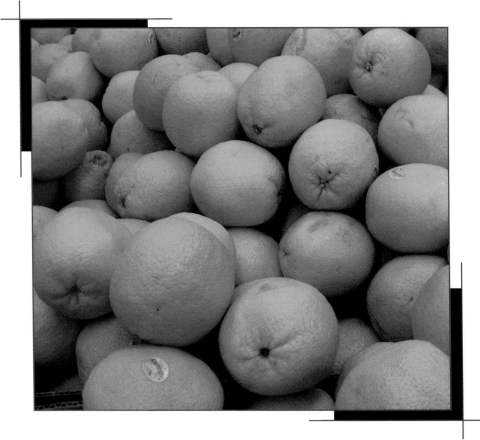

GRAPEFRUIT

Grapefruit is a subtropical citrus tree grown for its bitter fruit, an 18th-century hybrid first bred in Jamaica. When found in Barbados it was named the "forbidden fruit", it is also called the "shaddock", after its creator.

The fruit is yellow-orange skinned and largely oblate, and ranges in diameter from 10–15 cm. Grapefruit comes in many varieties, determinable by color, which is caused by the pigmentation of the fruit in respect of both its state of ripeness and genetic bent. The most popular varieties cultivated today are red, white, and pink hues, referring to the inside, pulp color of the fruit. The family of flavors range from highly acidic and somewhat bitter to sweet and tart.

The US quickly became a major producer of the fruit, with orchards in Florida, Texas, Arizona, and California. In Spanish, the fruit is known as toronja or pomelo.

Therapeutic use: Grapefruits are rich in vitamin C, high fiber as well as other micro-nutrients and certain phyto-chemicals. The potassium and pectin, a soluble fiber in grapefruit is effective in lowering cholesterol levels. Beside this, the white pith contains pectin and bioflavonoids that are excellent antioxidant food. Bioflavonoids act as potent antioxidants which can bind to toxic metals and escort them out of the body.

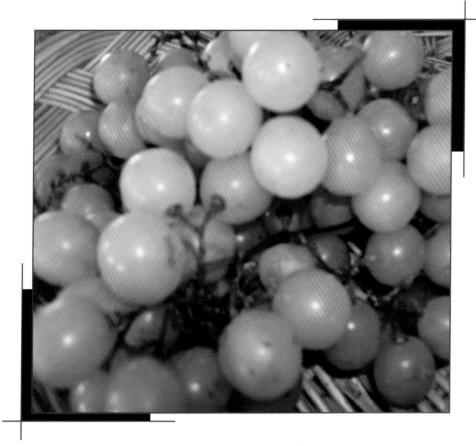

GRAPES

Grapes are small round or oval berries that feature semi-translucent flesh encased by a smooth skin. Some contain edible seeds while others are seedless. Like blueberries, grapes are covered by a protective, whitish bloom. Grapes that are eaten as is or used in a recipe are called table grapes as opposed to wine grapes (used in viniculture) or raisin grapes (used to make dried fruit).

Color, size, taste and physical characteristics differ amongst the varieties. Grapes come in a variety of colors including green, amber, red, blue-black, and purple. In general, whole grapes have a slightly crunchy texture and a dry, sweet and tart taste.

Currently, Italy, France, Spain, the United States, Mexico and Chile are among the largest commercial producers of grapes.

Therapeutic use: Grapes contain important vitamins such as vitamin A, B1, B2, B6 and C6. It also contain acids such as tartaric acids, malic acids, succinic, fumaric, glyceric, p-coumaric and caffeic acids. Beta-carotene, lycopene, ellagic acid, resveratrol and other sulphur compounds are found in grape skins. Grapes have important anti-oxidants such as anthocyanins, flavones, geraniol, linalol, nerol and tannins. Grapes contain all the necessary minerals such as calcium, chlorine, copper, fluorine, iron, magnesium, manganese, phosphorus, potassium, silicon and sulfur. Resveratrol, an important constituent of red wines, helps in the treatment of Alzheimer's disease. Grapes help fight neurodegenerative diseases.

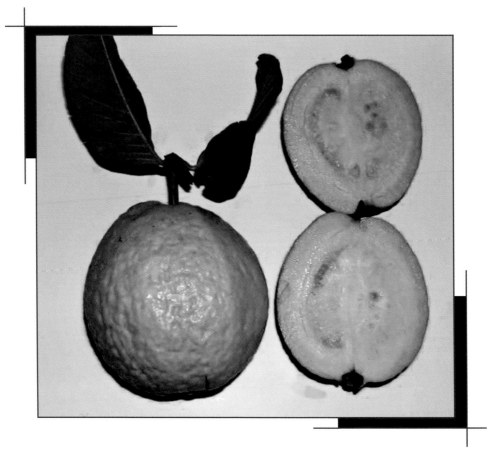

GUAPPLE

Guapple is a name given to this extra large, probably hybrid guava.

It weighs 400 to 1,000 grams per fruit. It produces thick and white-fleshed fruit but with a bland taste. The guapple's flesh is crispier since it is not as dense. The seeds are also less, but are far more distributed into the flesh, unlike the other guava which seeds are in a tight, compact ball that forms the fruit's core.

This fruit is eaten raw and can be processed into jelly, wine and guava jam preserves.

Therapeutic use: It is a good source of Vitamin C.

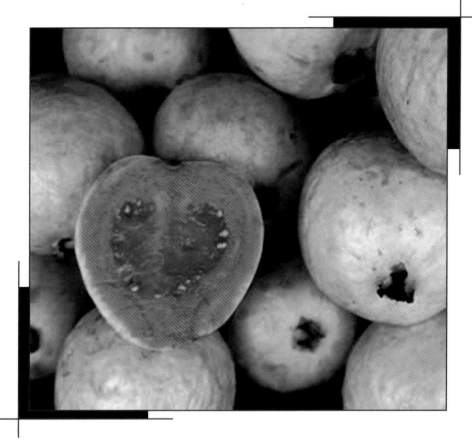

GUAVA

Guava (Psydium guajava), is also called guayabo, or guayavo, the fruit guayaba or guyava. The French call it goyave or goyavier; the Dutch, guyaba, goeajaaba; the Surinamese, guave or goejaba; and the Portuguese, goiaba or goaibeira. Hawaiians call it guava or kuawa. In Guam it is abas. In Malaya, it is generally known either as guava or jambu batu, but has also numerous dialectal names as it does in India, tropical Africa and the Philippines where the name, bayabas, is often applied. Various tribal names–pichi, posh, enandi, etc.–are employed among the Indians of Mexico and Central and South America.

Guava is a very aromatic fruit, with a pungent and penetrating odor, with lots of seeds (from 112 to 535) but great taste. It's native to Mexico and Central America but it's cultivated extensively in Florida and Hawaii.

Therapeutic use: Guava is often referred to as a superfruit containing large quantities of vitamins A and C, Omega 3 and 6 polyunsaturated fatty acids and high levels of dietary fibers.

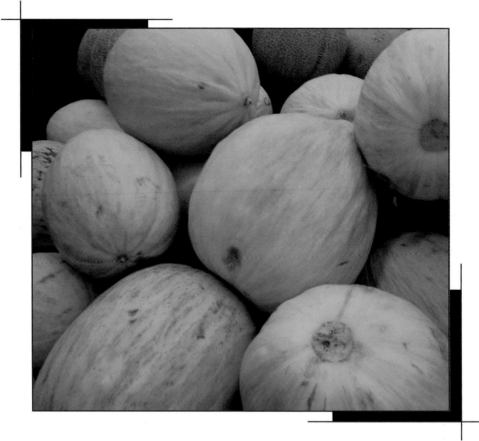

HONEYDEW MELON

Honeydew is a cultivar group of the muskmelon, Cucumis melo Inodorus group, which includes Crenshaw, casaba, Persian, winter, and other mixed melons. In China, honeydews are known as the Bailan melon.

The honeydew melon is almost perfectly round with a smooth, waxy white skin. The white can be slightly tinged with green, but not completely green. The rind should never be fuzzy. It should feel heavy, representing the density of the melon's inner flesh. It shouldn't feel completely hard on the outside, but the exterior should only barely yield to pressure from the hands. The inside view of the honeydew melon is undoubtedly attractive. When you cut it in half, you'll note its light green flesh, and a layer of seeds. These are easily scooped out with a spoon. You can merely eat the honeydew in slices, since it has a sweet and mild, melon flavor, or it can be cut into cubes to add to salads.

Therapeutic use: Honeydew melon has some nutritional value, especially in its Vitamin C content and is a fair source of protein.

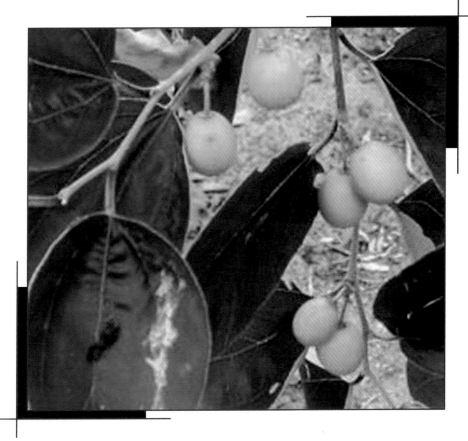

INDIAN JUJUBE

Indian Jujube (Zizyphus mauritiana), also called jujube, Chinese date or tsao, is native from Southern China to India but can be found in many other warmer countries. It differs from its more popular cousin, Chinese jujube, which is the hardier species that`s grown in cooler countries.

Depending on the various cultivars, it can be round, oval or oblong. The immature jujube is green, ripens to yellowish-green. It will turn fully brown or red when mature and starts to wrinkle when overripes.

It can be eaten whole, minus the single stone, at any of the ripening stages. Crisp, mildly sweet to astringent when green to yellow but soft, sweet and mealy when it ripens. It is usually smaller and not as sweet as the common(Chinese) jujubes.

Therapeutic use: Tests indicate that it is very high in vitamin C content. The fruit has been used medicinally for millennia by many cultures. One of its most popular uses is as a tea for sore throat

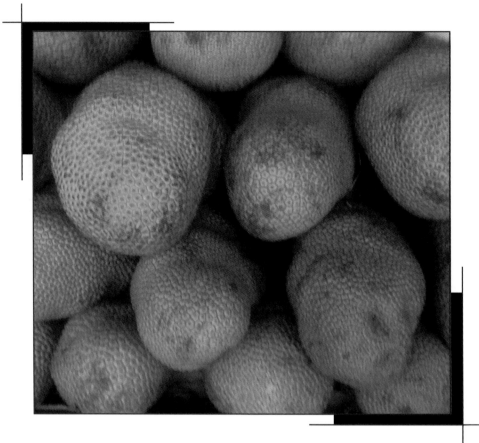

JACKFRUIT

Jackfruit (Artocarpus heterophyllus or Artocarpus heterophylla) is a species of tree in the mulberry family (Moraceae). It`s the largest tree borne fruit in the world. The fruits can reach 36 kg (80 lbs) in weight and up to 90 cm (36 in) long and 50 cm (20 in) in diameter.

The jackfruit is something of an acquired taste, but it is very popular in many parts of the world. The sweet yellow flesh around the seeds is about 3–5 mm thick and has a taste similar to that of pineapple, but milder and less juicy.

The jackfruit (not to be confused with the Durian fruit) is native to India, Bangladesh, Nepal and Sri Lanka. It is also possibly native to the Malay Peninsula, although it may have been introduced there by humans. It is commercially grown and sold in South, Southeast Asia and northern Australia. It is also grown in parts of Hawaii, Brazil, Suriname, Madagascar, and in islands of the West Indies such as Jamaica and Trinidad.

Therapeutic use: Jackfruit is rich in potassium, vitamin C, isoflavones and has been found to be helpful in the lowering of blood pressure. It contains phytonutrients, with health benefits ranging from anti-cancer to antihypertensive. Jackfruit is known to contain anti-ulcer properties and is also good for those suffering from indigestion. Boasting of anti-ageing properties, the fruit can help slow down the degeneration of cells and make the skin look young and supple. It serves as a good supply of proteins, carbohydrates and vitamins, for the human body. If you are suffering from constipation, regular consumption of the fruit will surely prove beneficial.

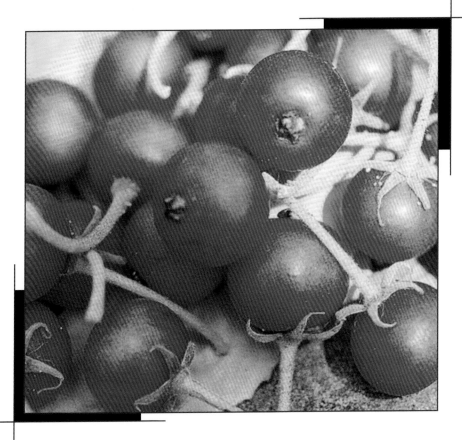

JAMAICAN CHERRY

Jamaican cherry (Muntingia calabura) is a small, round, green turning red when ripe fruit. These cherries are very sweet. The sweetness brings with it an excellent taste, because it has a lovely fragrance that makes people keep on eating them. These cherries are often eaten by children because they taste quite like cotton candy. They are just delicious. In fact, they are so delicious you might become addicted to eating them.

Also called Japanese cherry, Buah ceri/Kerukup Siam (Malay), aratilis (Philippines).

Fruits are eaten fresh, also made into jams and used in tarts.

This fruit is native to southern Mexico, Central America, tropical South America, the Great Antilles, St. Vincent and Trinidad. Widely introduced to almost all tropical regions.

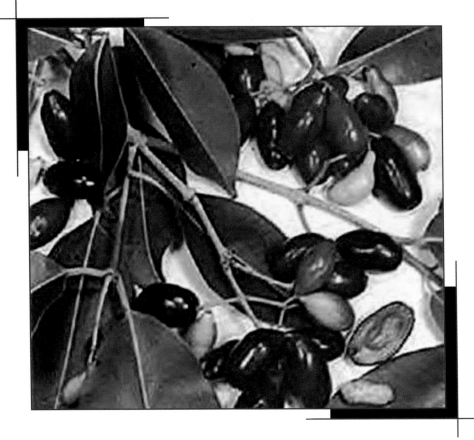

JAVA PLUM, JAMUN or DUHAT

Java Plum (Sizygium cumini), also known as Jamun, Nerale Hannu, Njaval, Jamlang, Jambolan, Black Plum, Damson Plum, Duhat Plum, Jambolan Plum, Jambul, and Portuguese Plum, is native to Bangladesh, India, Pakistan and Indonesia. It is also grown in other areas of southern Asia including Philippines, Myanmar and Afghanistan.

The fruit is oblong, ovoid, starts green and turns pink to shining crimson black as it matures. A variant of the tree produces white colored fruit. The fruit has a combination of sweet, mildly sour and astringent flavor and tends to color the tounge purple. Wine and vinegar are also made from the fruit.

Therapeutic use: It is a healthy fruit with absolutely no trace of sucrose and therefore the only fruit with minimum calories and a rich source of vitamin A and C. The juice of the fruit is extremely soothing and has a cooling effect, helping in the proper functioning of the digestive system.

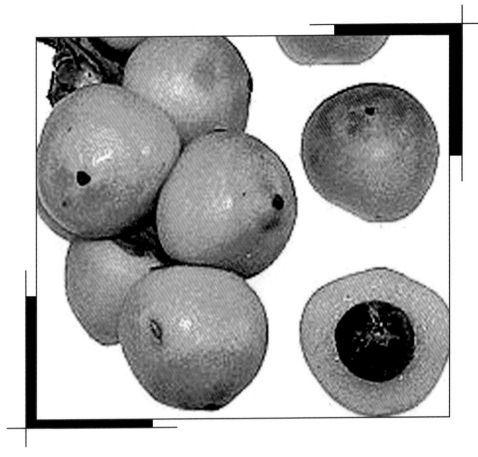

JELLY PALM FRUIT

Jelly palm fruit (Butia capitata), also called pindo palm and wine palm, is a South American monoecious palm native to Brazil.

The large cluster of yellowish-orange drupes is produced on a stalk near the base of the curved leaves. The one-inch, yellow to orange-colored fruits are round to oval-shaped, and hang in large sprays from the tree. Each fruit contains a single seed. The sweet-tart flavor is reminiscent of both apricots and a pineapple-banana mixture.

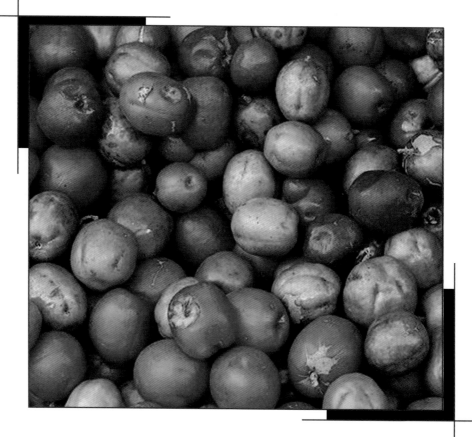

JOCOTE, RED MOMBIN, PURPLE MOMBIN

Jocote (Spondias purpurea) is a species native to tropical regions of the Americas. Other common names include Red Mombin, Purple Mombin, or Hog Plum, ciruela in Spanish, siniguelas in Philippines.

The fruit is an edible oval drupe, 3-5 cm long and 2-3.5 cm broad, ripening red (occasionally yellow) and containing a single large seed.

The fruits are often eaten ripe, with or without the skin. It is sometimes eaten unripe with salt.

It is now widely cultivated in tropical regions throughout the world for its edible fruit, and is also naturalised in some areas, including the Philippines and Nigeria. Numerous cultivars have been selected for fruit quality. It is also abundant in Central America.

Therapeutic use: In Mexico, the fruits are regarded as diuretic and antispasmodic. The fruit decoction is used to bathe wounds and heal sores in the mouth. A syrup prepared from the fruit is taken to overcome chronic diarrhea.

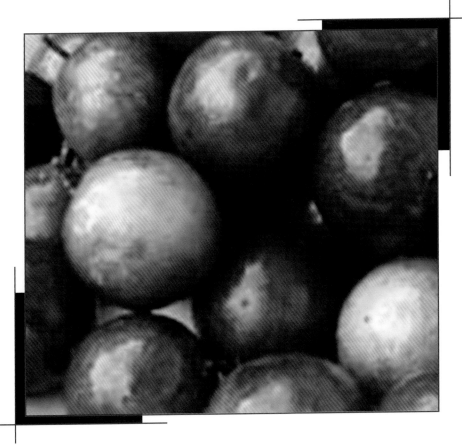

KALUMPIT

Kalumpit (Terminalia edulis Blanco) is a fruit that comes from a large tree that can grow up to 25 meters. It is a very common and widely distributed species in primary forests at low altitudes from Luzon to southern Mindanao in Philippines. It is also reported from Java.

The fruit is about 3cm wide, smooth and when fully ripe turns to a nice burgundy red. Fruit is fleshy and acid. Besides being eaten raw, also makes a good preserve and used to flavor and age lambanog (coconut liquor).

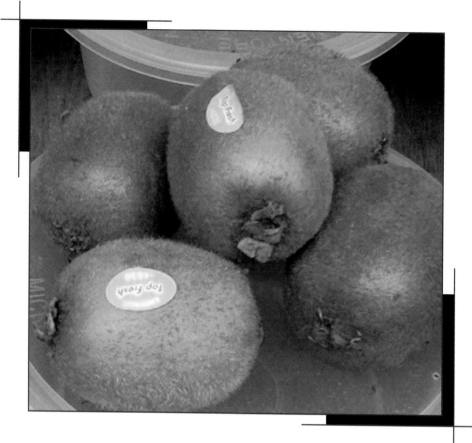

KIWI FRUIT

Kiwi fruit is the edible berry of a cultivar group of the woody vine Actinidia deliciosa and hybrids between this and other species in the genus Actinidia. The Actinidia is native to South of China.

Also known as Chinese gooseberry, today is a commercial crop in several countries, mainly in Italy, China, and New Zealand.

This fruit consists of a hairy, brown peel containing green flesh, with white pulp in the center, surrounded by black, edible seeds. The fruit has a sweet taste, similar to a mixture of banana, pineapple and strawberry. Kiwi fruits are native to China, where they were called "macaque peach".

Therapeutic use: Nutrition-wise, kiwi fruits contain about as much potassium as bananas, and also contain 1.5 times the DRI for Vitamin C. It is also rich in Vitamins A and E, and its black seeds can be crushed to produce kiwi fruit oil, which is very rich in Alpha-Linoleic Acid.

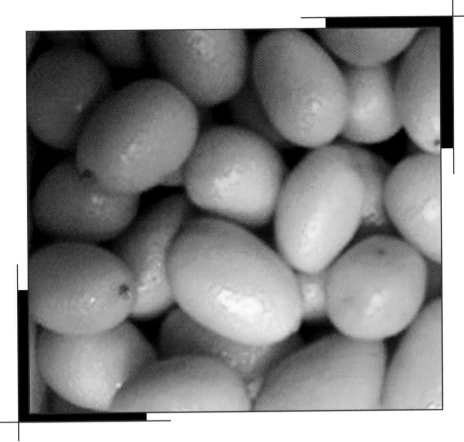

KUMQUATS

Kumquats (Fortunella japonica), also called kinkan, have been called "the little germs of the citrus family". Although kumquat trees are native to, and prevalent in Asia-specifically in China and Indochina -- they are also cultivated in Japan and in the United States, in warmer states such as California and Florida.

Kumquats are small, edible fruits that look similar to oranges. These fruits are extremely juicy and tasty and usually have a sweet outer skin accompanied by a tart, inner flesh. An exception to this is the Meiwa kumquat. This kumquat type has a sweet outer skin and a sweet inner flesh. You can easily identify a kumquat by its bright skin color, which is either orange or yellow. Additionally, kumquats are approximately 1 to 1 1/2 inches in length and are either oval or round in shape depending on the type of kumquat grown. For instance, the Nagami kumquat is oval shaped and has a yellow skin. Meanwhile, the Marumi kumquat has a round shape and an orange colored skin. While the most common use for the kumquat fruit is to eat it whole, as is, other popular uses for the fruit include adding pieces of it to fruit salads or to dessert recipes. Kumquats are also used to make jellies, jams and marmalades and are often pickled, whole or preserved in syrups for future use.

Therapeutic use: Kumquats are diverse fruits that also offer many nutritional benefits. They are cholesterol, fat, and sodium free and provide a good source of fiber and of the vitamins A and C. Kumquats contain traces of calcium and iron. For those on a diet, approximately eight kumquats contain 100 calories. Thus, they offer a sweet alternative to other less healthy snack foods.

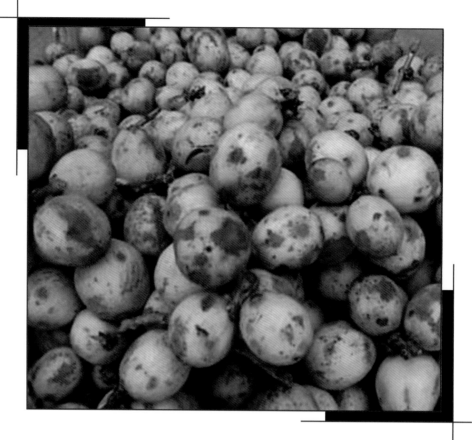

LANGSAT, LANZONES

Langsat (Lansium duranum), also known as Lanzones in the Philippines, was originally native to the Malaysian peninsula. It is known variously as langsat (Malay); lansones, lansa, buahan, langseh, langsep, lanzon, lanzone, lansones (Filipino); langsad (for the type of which its skin is quite sticky to the fruit), longkong (for the type of which the skin is easily peeled off without milky latex) (Thai); duku, kokosan (Indonesian), Gadu Guda (Sri Lanka), lòn bon and bòn bon (Vietnamese).

Agriculturally, the tree is grown throughout the entire Southeast asian region, ranging from Southern India to the Philippines for its fruit. Within mainland Asia, the tree is cultivated in Thailand, Vietnam and India, as well as its native Malaysia. Outside the region, it has also been successfully transplanted and introduced to Hawaii and Surinam.

Fruits are ovoid, roundish orbs, usually found in clusters of two to thirty fruits. Each round fruit is covered by yellowish, thick, leathery skin. Underneath the skin, the fruit is divided into five or six slices of translucent, juicy flesh. The flesh is slightly acidic in taste, although ripe specimens are sweeter. Green seeds are present in around half of the segments, usually taking up a small portion of the segment although some seeds take up the entire segment's volume. In contrast with the sweet-sour flavor of the fruit's flesh, the seeds are extremely bitter. The sweet juicy flesh contains sucrose, fructose, and glucose.

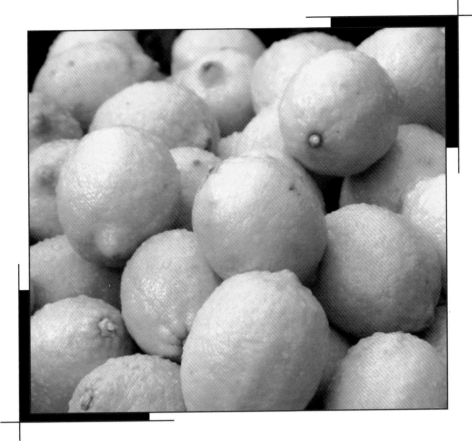

LEMON

Lemon (Citrus limon), is used for both culinary and nonculinary purposes throughout the world. The fruit is used primarily for its juice, though the pulp and rind (zest) are also used, primarily in cooking and baking. Lemon juice is about 5% (approximately 0.3 mole per liter) citric acid, which gives lemon a tart taste, and a pH of 2 to 3. This makes lemon juice an inexpensive, readily available acid for use in educational science experiments. Because of the tart flavor, many lemon-flavored drinks and candies are available on the market, including lemonade.

Among the world's leading lemon growers and exporters are Italy, Spain, Greece, Turkey, Cyprus, Lebanon, South Africa and Australia. Lemons can be grown only at medium and high elevations in the Philippines.

Therapeutic use: Lemons and limes are an excellent source of vitamin C, one of the most important antioxidants in nature.

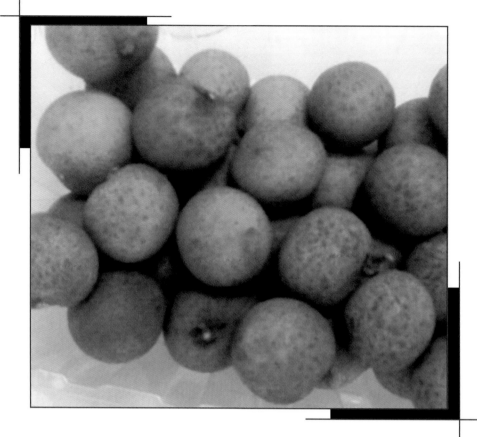

LONGAN

Longan "dragon eye" (Dimocarpus longan) is a tropical tree native to southern China. It is also found in Southeast Asia. It is also called guiyuan in Chinese, lengkeng in Indonesia, mata kucing (literally "cat's eye") in Malaysia, named long nhãn in Vietnamese- (literally "dragon's eyes"), Mora in Sinhalese (Sri Lanka) and also "longan" in Tagalog.

The longan ("dragon eyes") is so named because of the fruit's resemblance to an eyeball when it is shelled (the black seed shows through the translucent flesh like a pupil/iris). The seed is small, round and hard.

The fruit is edible, and is often used in East Asian soups, snacks, desserts, and sweet-and-sour foods, either fresh or dried, sometimes canned with syrup in supermarkets.

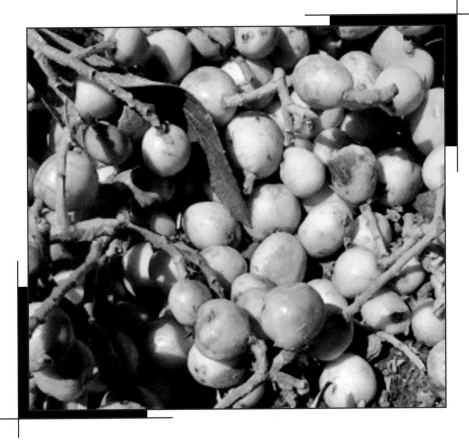

LOQUATS

Loquat (Eriobotrya japonica) is a fruit indigenous to southeastern China. It has also been known as Japanese meddler. It was introduced into Japan and became naturalised there in very early times, and has been cultivated there for over 1,000 years. It has also become naturalised in India, the whole Mediterranean Basin and many other areas. Chinese immigrants are presumed to have carried the loquat to Hawaii.

Loquat fruits, growing in clusters, are oval, rounded or pear-shaped, 3-5 cm long, with a smooth or downy, yellow or orange, sometimes red-blushed skin. The succulent, tangy flesh is white, yellow or orange and sweet to subacid or acid, depending on the cultivar. Each fruit contains five ovules, of which one to five mature into large brown seeds. The skin, though thin, can be peeled off manually if the fruit is ripe.

The loquat is comparable with its distant relative, the apple, in many aspects, with a high sugar, acid and pectin content. It is eaten as a fresh fruit and mixes well with other fruits in fresh fruit salads or fruit cups. Firm, slightly immature fruits are best for making pies or tarts. The fruits are also commonly used to make jam, jelly, and chutney, and are often served poached in light syrup.

Therapeutic use: This fruit is very low in Saturated Fat, Cholesterol and Sodium. It is also a good source of Dietary Fiber, Vitamin B6, Potassium and Manganese, and a very good source of Vitamin A.

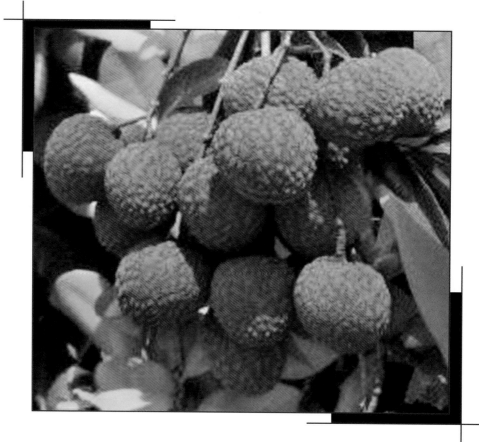

LYCHEE

Lychee (Litchi chinensis) or laichi and lichu is the sole member of the genus Litchi in the soapberry family Sapindaceae. It is a tropical fruit tree. It is primarily found in China, India, Madagascar, Nepal, Bangladesh, Pakistan, southern and central Taiwan, northern Vietnam, Indonesia, Thailand, the Philippines, Southern Africa and Mexico. It is a fragranced fruit with a sweet taste.

The fruit is a drupe, 3–4 cm long and 3 cm in diameter. The outside is covered by a pink-red, roughly-textured rind that is inedible but easily removed. They are eaten in many different dessert dishes. The inside consists of a layer of sweet, translucent white flesh, rich in vitamin C, with a texture somewhat similar to that of a grape only much less moist. The edible flesh consists of a highly developed aril enveloping the seed. The center contains a single glossy brown nut-like seed, 2 cm long and 1–1.5 cm in diameter. The seed, similar to a buckeye seed, is not poisonous but should not be eaten.

Therapeutic use: This fruit is low in Saturated Fat, and very low in Cholesterol and Sodium. It is also a good source of Copper, and a very good source of Vitamin C.

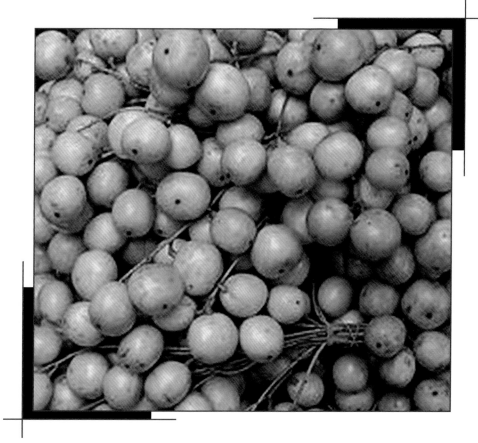

MAFAI, BURMESE GRAPE

Mafai or Burmese grape (Baccaurea ramiflora), also called Mafai, is an oval, colored yellowish, pinkish to bright red or purple fruit, 2.5-3.5 cm in diameter, glaborous, with 2-4 large purple-red seed, with white aril.

The fruit is usually eaten fresh, stewed or made into wine, the seeds are edible as well.

It is found throughout Asia, most commonly cultivated in India and Malaysia.

Therapeutic use: It is also used medicinally to treat skin diseases.

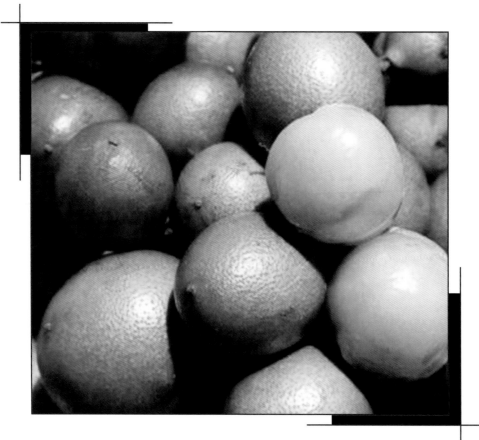

MAMONCILLO

Mamoncillo fruit (Melicoccus bijugatus), also known as mamón, chenet (in Trinidad and Tobago), guaya, gnep, ginep, skinnip (in Jamaica, St. Kitts) genip, guinep, ginnip, kenèp (in Guyana, Haiti, Belize, Bahamas) quenepa, genepa, xenepa (in Puerto Rico), and Spanish lime, limoncillo (in the Dominican Republic), is a fruit in the soapberry family Sapindaceae, native or naturalised over a wide area of the American tropics including Central America, Mexico, Colombia, Venezuela, Dominican Republic, Guyana, Suriname and the Caribbean.

The fruit is an ovoid, green fruit, which grow in bunches. For eating out-of-hand, the rind is merely torn open at the stem end and the pulp-coated seed is squeezed into the mouth, the juice being sucked from the pulp until there is nothing left of it but the fiber. With fruits that have non-adherent pulp, the latter may be scraped from the seed and utilized to make pie-filling, jam, marmalade or jelly, but this entails much work for the small amount of edible material realized. More commonly, the peeled fruits are boiled and the resulting juice is prized for cold drinks. In Colombia, the juice is canned commercially.

The seeds are eaten after roasting. Indians of the Orinoco consume the cooked seeds as a substitute for cassava.

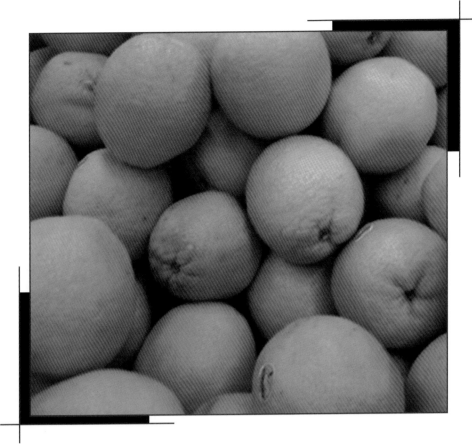

MANDARIN ORANGE

Mandarin orange (Citrus reticulata), also known as mandarin or mandarine, is a small citrus tree with fruit resembling the orange. In the Philippines, all mandarin oranges are called naranjita. Spanish speaking people in the American tropics call them mandarina.

The mandarin orange is considered a native of south-eastern Asia and the Philippines. It is most abundantly grown in Japan, southern China, India, and the East Indies, and is esteemed for home consumption in Australia.

The fruit is oblate, the peel bright-orange or red-orange when ripe, loose, separating easily from the segments. Seeds are small, pointed at one end, green inside.

Mandarin oranges of all kinds are primarily eaten out-of-hand, or the sections are utilized in fruit salads, gelatins, puddings, or on cakes. Very small types are canned in syrup.

Therapeutic use: This fruit is very low in Saturated Fat, Cholesterol and Sodium. It is also a good source of Thiamin and Potassium, and a very good source of Vitamin A and Vitamin C.

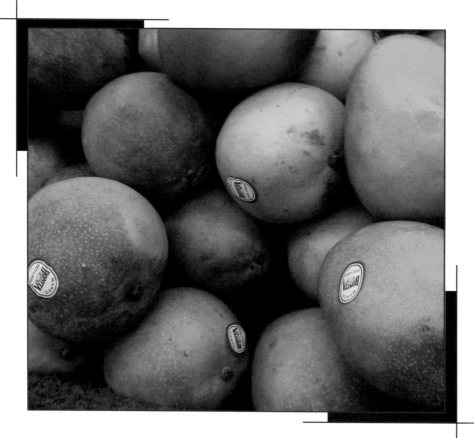

MANGO

Mangoes (Mangifera indica), also called mangot, manga, mangou, is native to southern Asia, especially Burma and eastern India. Cultivated in many tropical regions and distributed widely in the world, mango is one of the most extensively exploited fruits for food, juice, flavor, fragrance and color, making it a common ingredient in new functional foods often called superfruits.

The ripe fruit is variable in size and color, and may be yellow, orange, red or green when unripe, depending on the cultivar. When ripe, the unpeeled fruit gives off a distinctive resinous sweet smell. In its center is a single flat oblong seed that can be fibrous or hairy on the surface, depending on the cultivar. Inside the seed coat 1–2 mm thick is a thin lining covering a single embryo, 4–7 cm long, 3–4 cm wide, and 1 cm thick.

A ripe mango is sweet, with a unique taste that nevertheless varies from variety to variety. The texture of the flesh varies between cultivars, some having a soft, pulpy texture similar to an over-ripe plum, while others have firmer flesh like a cantaloupe or avocado. In some cultivars, the flesh has a fibrous texture.

Therapeutic use: Mangoes are high in Vitamin C, Vitamin B6, Potassium, Copper and Vitamin A. Mangoes also contain several important phytochemicals including: Cryptoxanthin, Lutein, Gallic Acid and Anacardic acid. High in fiber, virtually fat-free, and mangoes contain numerous vitamins. Mangoes also contain beta-carotene which may help slow the aging process, reduce the risk of certain forms of cancer, improve lung function, and reduce complications associated with diabetes.

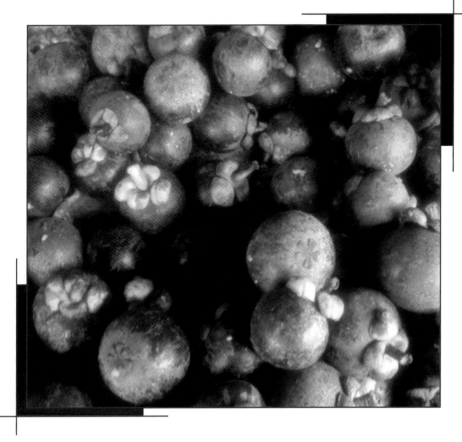

MANGOSTEEN

Mangosteen (Garcinia mangostana) is a tropical fruit that is commonly grown in hot and humid climates of Southeast Asia such as Thailand, Vietnam, Indonesia, and Singapore.

The color of the fruit is usually dark purple which grows to a diameter of about 2 to 3 inches. Its size is most likely that of a small peach or apple. However, mangosteens are not related to mangos.

The rind of the edible fruit is deep reddish purple when ripe. Botanically an aril, the fragrant edible flesh can be described as sweet and tangy, citrusy with peach flavor and texture.

Therapeutic use: Mangosteen is high in vitamins A and C, catechins (potent antioxidants), polysaccharides, and stibenes (inorganic gas). It has long been recognized in Asia that mangosteen has powerful anti-inflammatory properties and is effective in treating eczema and other skin conditions such as psoriasis.

In the Caribbean, mangosteen tea is used as a tonic for fatigue and low energy. Brazilians use a similar tea as a deworming agent and digestive aid. In Venezuela, parasitic skin infections are treated with poultices of the fruit rind, while Filipinos employ a fruit extract to control fever.

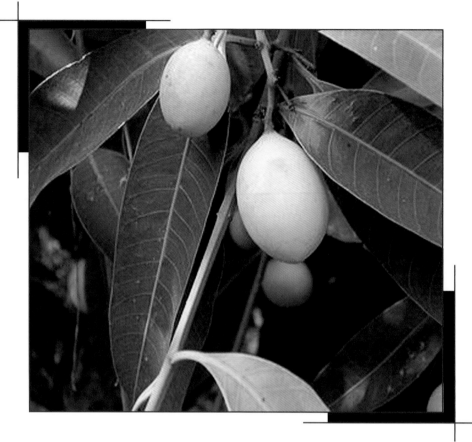

MAPRANG

Maprang (Bouea gandaria Blume), also called marian plum is a green to orange-yellow resembling a mango fruit, but slightly smaller. The tree belongs to the same family as the mango, Anacardiaceae, and it has similar leaves, albeit smaller.

The fruits are eaten fresh. Flavor is sour to sweetish.

It is native to Malaysia and Western Java. The maprang is commercially grown in Thailand, Indonesia and Malaysia.

Therapeutic use: It is high in beta carotene and anti-oxidant properties known to inhibit cancers and other diseases.

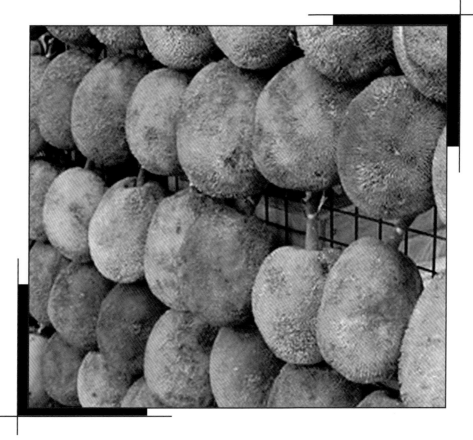

MARANG

Marang (Artocarpus odoratissimus) - also called Johey Oak, Madang and Tarap - is native to Borneo. It is closely related to the jackfruit, cempedak and breadfruit.

The fruit has a strong scent and is considered superior in flavor to both Jackfruit and Cempedak. The appearance of the fruit can be regarded as an intermediate shape between the jackfruit and the breadfruit. The fruit is round to oblong, 15-20 cm long and 13 cm broad, and weighing about 1 kg. The thick rind is covered with soft, broad spines. They become hard and brittle as the fruit matures. The fruit does not fall to the ground when ripe. It may be harvested while still hard, and left to ripen until soft. Marangs change color to greenish yellow when ripe. The ripe fruit is opened by cutting the rind around, twisting and gently pulling. The interior of the fruit is somewhat similar to the jackfruit's, but the color is white and the flesh is usually softer. The core is relatively large, but there are far fewer "rags" and less non-edible parts. Arils are white and the size of a grape, each containing a 15×8 mm seed. Once opened, the marang should be consumed quickly (in a few hours), as it loses flavor rapidly and fruit oxidizes. The seeds are also edible after boiling or roasting.

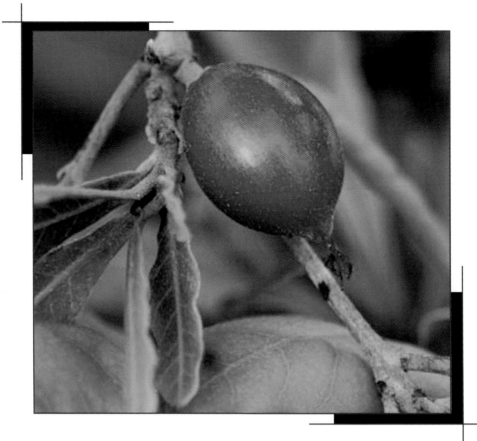

MIRACLE FRUIT

Miracle fruit, or miracle berry plant (Synsepalum dulcificum), produces berries that, when eaten, cause sour foods (such as lemons and limes) subsequently consumed to taste sweet.

The berry contains an active glycoprotein molecule, with some trailing carbohydrate chains, called miraculin. When the fleshy part of the fruit is eaten, this molecule binds to the tongue's taste buds, causing sour foods to taste sweet. While the exact cause for this change is unknown, one hypothesis is that the effect may be caused if miraculin works by distorting the shape of sweetness receptors "so that they become responsive to acids, instead of sugar and other sweet things". This effect lasts 15-30 minutes.

In Japan, miracle fruit is popular among diabetics and dieters. Miracle fruit is available as freeze-dried granules or in tablets — this form has a longer shelf life than fresh fruit. Tablets are made from compressed freeze-dried fruit which causes the texture to be clearly visible even in tablet form.

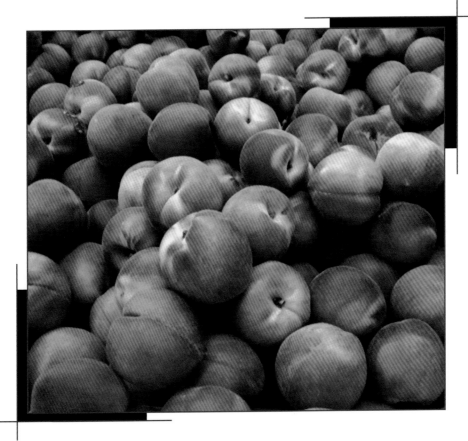

NECTARINE

Nectarine (Prunus persica var. nectarina) is virtually identical to the fruit we call peaches, except for one noticeable feature. The skin of most peaches contains fuzz, while the skin of nectarines is smooth. The same mutation responsible for the smooth skin is also responsible for the spicier taste and slightly smaller size of nectarines. Nectarines and peaches both grow from the same parent peach trees, which have been known to produce examples of both fruits at the same time. Essentially there are no nectarine trees, only peach trees with a genetic mutation.

Nectarines can be traced back to ancient China, where peaches and nectarines were very symbolic and revered fruits.

Nectarines taste best consumed "warm" from the tree. Often jam is made out of it because they can't be stored fresh. Nectarines are mostly eaten with the skin.

Therapeutic use: Nectarines provide an excellent amount of Vitamin A and a significant amount of Vitamin C.

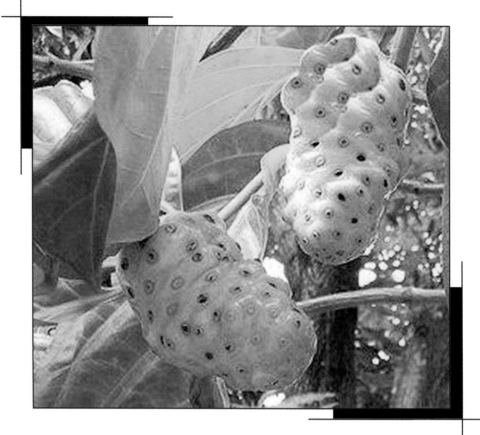

NONI

Noni (Morinda citrifolia), commonly known as great morinda, Indian mulberry, Mekudu (Malaysia), beach mulberry, Tahitian noni, cheese fruit, or noni (Hawaii), is native to Southeast Asia but has been extensively spread throughout the Indian subcontinent, Pacific islands, French Polynesia, Puerto Rico and Dominican Republic. Tahiti remains the most prominent growing location.

The fruit is a multiple fruit that has a pungent odor when ripening, and is hence also known as cheese fruit or even vomit fruit. It is oval and reaches 4–7 centimetres (1.6–2.8 in) in size. At first green, the fruit turns yellow then almost white as it ripens. It contains many seeds. Southeast Asians and Australian Aborigines consume the fruit raw with salt or cook it with curry. The seeds are edible when roasted.

Therapeutic use: Noni has been reported to have a range of health benefits for colds, cancer, diabetes, asthma, hypertension, pain, skin infection, high blood pressure, mental depression, atherosclerosis and arthritis. The noni contain the antibacterial compounds in the fruits (acubin, L-asperuloside and alizarin) and roots (anthrauinones). Noni contains scopoletin which inhibits the growth of Escherichia coli, which is responsible for intestinal infections, and Heliobacter pylori, which causes ulcers. Damnacanthal, which is found in the noni roots, inhibits the tyrosine kinase and gives noni antitumor activity.

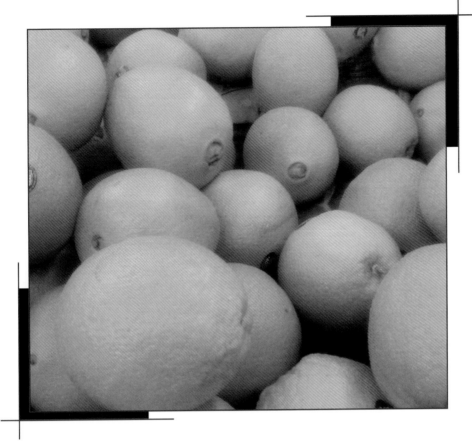

ORANGE

Orange—specifically, the sweet orange—is the citrus Citrus ×sinensis and its fruit. The orange is a hybrid of ancient cultivated origin, possibly between pomelo (Citrus maxima) and tangerine (Citrus reticulata). The orange fruit is a hesperidium, a type of berry. Oranges originated in Southeast Asia.

Like all citrus fruits, the orange is acidic, with a pH level of around 2.5-3; depending on the age, size and variety of the fruit. Although this is not, on average, as strong as the lemon, it is still quite strong on the pH scale – as strong as vinegar.

Oranges grown for commercial production are generally grown in groves and are produced throughout the world. The top three orange-producing countries are Brazil, the United States, and Mexico.

Therapeutic use: This fruit is very low in Saturated Fat, Cholesterol and Sodium. It is also a good source of Thiamin, Folate and Potassium, and a very good source of Dietary Fiber and Vitamin C.

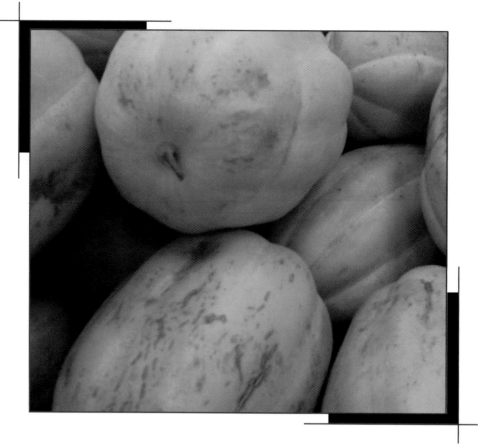

ORIENTAL MELON

Oriental Melon Fruits have smooth, golden skin and crisp, sweet white flesh with the sugar content at 12 brix. The oblong-shaped melon is 4-6 inches long and 3-4 inches wide, 350 grams in weight. Plant grows vigorously in warm climates. This melon is very prolific and is very popular in Taiwan, Korea and Japan.

Therapeutic use: The Oriental melon contains Vitamin E and calcium in quantity. Also, it contains considerable amount of water, which stimulates urination.

This fruit is effective to discharge phlegm, cure palsy, jaundice, constipation etc. It also has anti-cancer materials. In summer when people sweat a lot, this fruit is good for quenching the thirst.

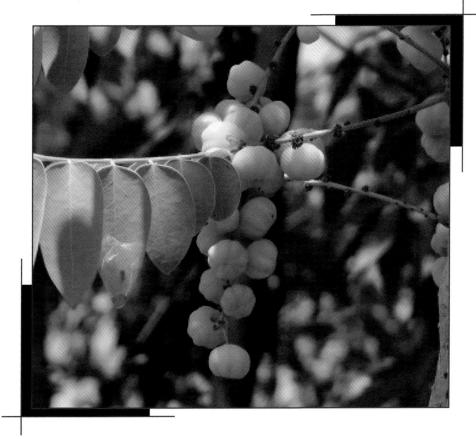

OTAHEITE GOOSEBERRY

Otaheite gooseberry, (Phyllanthus acidus), is totally unlike a gooseberry except for its acidity. This fruit is variously known as Malay gooseberry, country gooseberry, kemangor (Malaya); cherme (Java); chum ruot (Vietnam); mayom (Thailand); mak-nhom (Laos); star gooseberry, West India gooseberry, jumbling, chalmeri, harpharori (India); iba (Philippines); ciruela (Mexico), wild plum (Belize); jumbling (Jamaica) pimiento or guinda (El salvador); grosella ((Costa Rica, Cuba); groselha (Brazil).

The fruits are small, white to slightly yellow colored borne in great abundance, with a crunchy, juicy, acidic flavored pulp. Often the fruit is cooked with sugar, upon which the pulp and juice turns bright red. Common uses for the resulting fruit mixture are to prepare beverages or use as sauce.

Native to Madagascar, but was spread long ago by humans throughout much of India, Southeast Asia, and some Pacific islands.

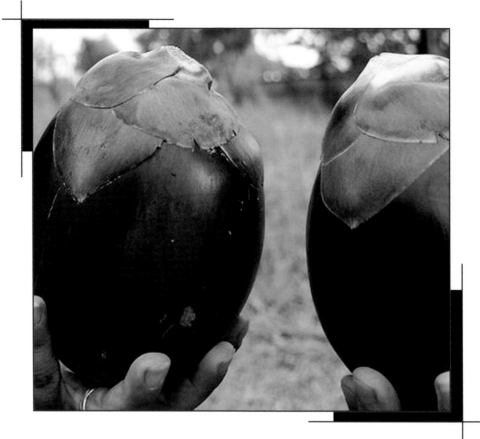

PALMYRA PALM FRUIT

Palmyra Palm Fruit (Borassus flabellifer) is also known as Fan palm, Brab tree, Todd palm, and Tala palm. In Hindi and Bengali, it is called Tal, Talgach and Tarkajhar. It is known as Pannei in Tamil language. This is found in the drier areas of Sri Lanka, Burma and also in most of the tropical countries. Though India is not the native of this tree, it is now expansively cultivated here.

The fruits are eaten roasted or raw, and the young jellylike seeds are eaten. A sugary sap, called Toddy, can be obtained from the young inflorescene, either male or female ones. The toddy is fermented to make a beverage called arrack, or it is concentrated to a crude sugar called jaggery/palm sugar.

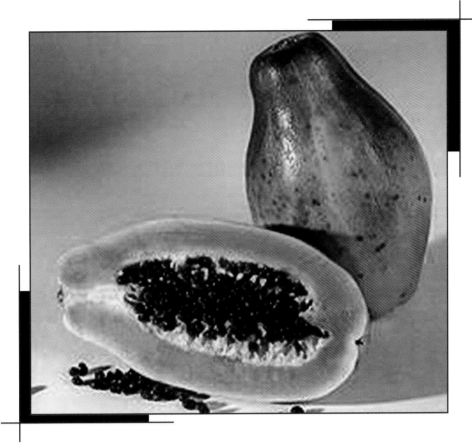

PAPAYA

Papaya (Carica papaya), also called Papaw or Paw Paw (Australia), Mamao (Brazil), Tree Melon, is believed to be native to southern Mexico and neighbor Central America. It is now present in every tropical and subtropical country.

There are two types of papayas, Hawaiian and Mexican. The Hawaiian varieties are the papayas commonly found in supermarkets. These pear-shaped fruit generally weigh about 1 pound and have yellow skin when ripe. The flesh is bright orange or pinkish, depending on variety, with small black seeds clustered in the center. The ripe fruit is usually eaten raw, without the skin or seeds. The unripe green fruit of papaya can be eaten cooked, usually in curries, salads and stews. It also has a relatively high amount of pectin, which can be used to make jellies. Mexican papayas are much larger than the Hawaiian types and may weight up to 10 pounds and be more than 15 inches long. The flesh may be yellow, orange or pink. The flavor is less intense than that the Hawaiian papaya but still is delicious and extremely enjoyable. A properly ripened papaya is juicy, sweetish and somewhat like a cantaloupe in flavor, although musky in some types. The fruit (and leaves) contain papain which helps digestion and is used to tenderize meat. The edible seeds have a spicy flavor somewhat reminiscent of black pepper.

Therapeutic use: This food is very low in Saturated Fat, Cholesterol and Sodium. It is also a good source of Dietary Fiber and Potassium, and a very good source of Vitamin A, Vitamin C and Folate.

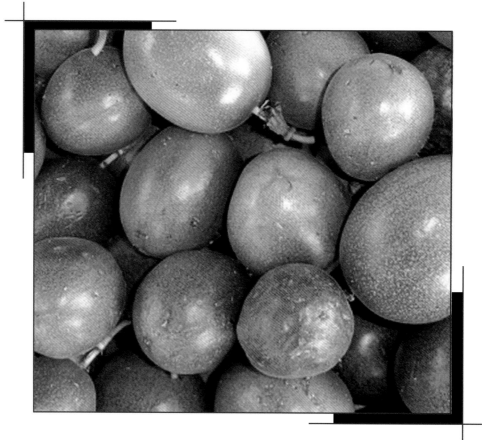

PASSION FRUIT

Passion fruit (Passiflora edulis), also called granadilla, maracuya , parcha (spanish), or maracujá (portuguese), is a plant cultivated commercially in frost-free areas for its fruit. It is native to South America and widely grown in India, New Zealand, the Caribbean, Brazil, Colombia, Ecuador, Indonesia, Peru, California, Florida, Hawaii, Australia, East Africa, Israel and South Africa.

The passion fruit is round to oval, yellow or dark purple at maturity, with a soft to firm, juicy interior filled with numerous seeds. The fruit can be grown to eat or for its juice, which is often added to other fruit juices to enhance aroma.

The two types of passion fruit have clearly differing exterior appearances. The bright yellow variety of passion fruit, which is also known as the Golden Passionfruit, can grow up to the size of a grapefruit, has a smooth, glossy, light and airy rind, and has been used as a rootstock for the purple passion fruit in Australia. The dark purple passion fruit is smaller than a lemon.

Therapeutic use: Fresh passion fruit is known to be high in vitamin A, potassium, and dietary fiber. The yellow variety is used for juice processing, while the purple variety is sold in fresh fruit markets. Passion fruit juice is a good source of ascorbic acid (vitamin C).

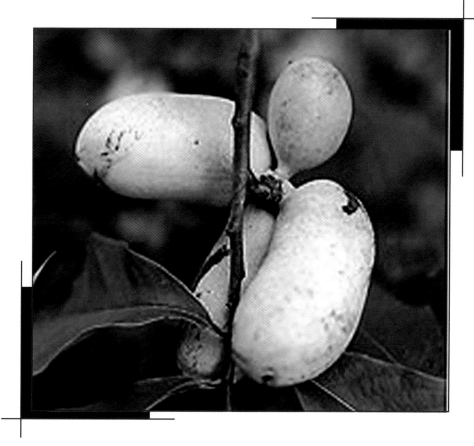

PAWPAW

Pawpaw fruit (Asimina triloba) is a large edible berry, 5 to 16cm long and 3 to 7cm broad, weighing from 20 to 500g, with numerous seeds; it is green when unripe, maturing to yellow or brown. It has a flavor somewhat similar to both banana and mango, varying significantly by cultivar, and has more protein than most fruits.

It is a genus of small clustered trees with large leaves and fruit, native to North America.

Pawpaw has numerous other common names, often very local, such as prairie banana, Indiana (Hoosier) banana, West Virginia banana, Kentucky banana, Michigan banana, Missouri banana, the poor man`s banana, and Ozark banana.

Therapeutic use: Pawpaws are very nutritious fruits. They are high in vitamin C, magnesium, iron, copper, and manganese. They are a good source of potassium and several essential amino acids, and they also contain significant amounts of riboflavin, niacin, calcium, phosphorus, and zinc.

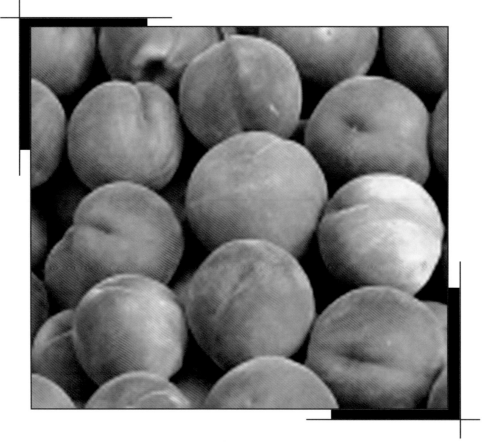

PEACH

Peach (Prunus persica) is known as a species of Prunus native to China that bears an edible juicy fruit also called a peach.

The fruit has yellow or whitish flesh, a delicate aroma, and a skin that is either velvety (peaches) or smooth (nectarines) in different cultivars. The flesh is very delicate and easily bruised in some cultivars, but is fairly firm in some commercial varieties, especially when green. The single, large seed is red-brown, oval shaped, approximately 1.3–2 cm long, and is surrounded by a wood-like husk. Peaches, along with cherries, plums and apricots, are stone fruits (drupes).

Important historical peach-producing areas are China, Iran, France, and the Mediterranean countries like Italy, Spain and Greece. More recently, the United States (where the three largest producing states are California, South Carolina, and Georgia), Canada (British Columbia), and Australia (the Riverland region) have also become important; peach growing in the Niagara Peninsula of Ontario, Canada, was formerly intensive but ended in 2008 when the last fruit cannery in Canada was closed by the proprietors.

Therapeutic use: A medium peach (75g), has 30 Cal, 7g of carbohydrate (6g sugars and 1g fiber), 1g of protein, 140mg of potassium, and 8% of the daily value (DV) for vitamin C.

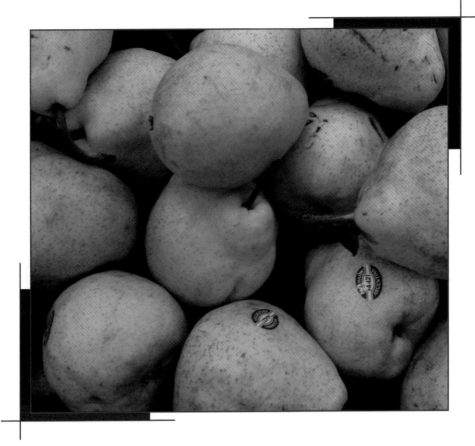

PEARS

Pear is an edible pomaceous fruit produced by a tree of genus Pyrus. The pear is classified within Maloideae, a subfamily within Rosaceae.

Pears have a distinctive bell shape fruit. Some pears have knobby lobes at the base of the fruit while others are smooth at the base. The skin of the fruit ranges in color from green, yellow, red, brown, pink, or a combination of these colors. Pear flesh is white and juicy and grainy in texture.

Pears are consumed fresh, canned, as juice, and dried. The juice can also be used in jellies and jams, usually in combination with other fruits or berries. Fermented pear juice is called perry.

Therapeutic use: Pears are rich in Vitamin A, Vitamin C, E1, copper and potassium. Pears are the least allergenic of all fruits. Because of this, it is sometimes used as the first juice introduced to infants.

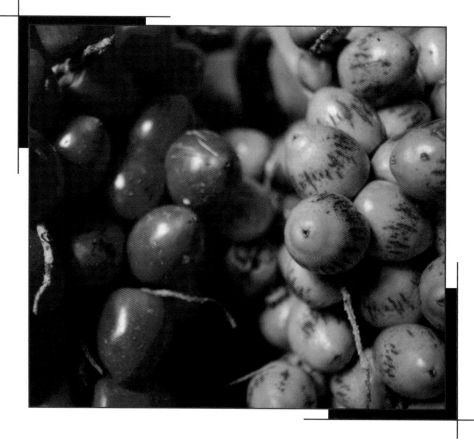

PEJIBAYE PALM FRUIT

Pejibaye (Bactris gasipaes), a relative of the coconut, grow in clusters on palm trees, like miniature coconuts.

The part that you eat would correspond to the fibrous husk, while the hard pejibaye seed, when cracked open, reveals a thin layer of bitter white meat around a hollow core. The bright orange or red pejibayes are delicious boiled in salted water, then peeled, halved and pitted and eaten alone or with mayonnaise. Their flavor is difficult to describe. They are not sweet, but more of a combination of chestnut and pumpkin with a thick, fibrous texture.

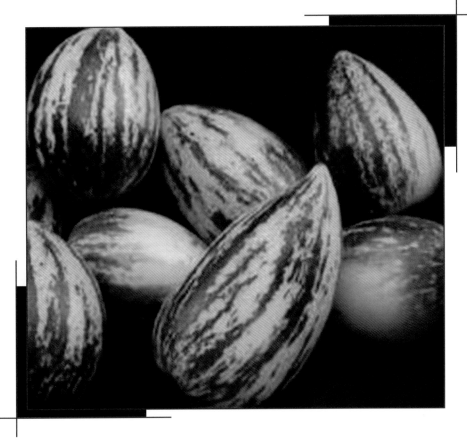

PEPINO

Pepino or pepino dulce (Solanum muricatum), is an exotic fruit that is produced from the pepino plant, which is a small bush that resembles a tomato vine and which grows to approximately three feet in height. Although it is native to South America, is it also grown in Australia, New Zealand, and in the United States, in California.

The pepino has a taste that is similar to a cucumber, cantaloupe, and a honeydew melon. Because of this, other common names for the pepino include melon shrub, tree melon, mellowfruit, pear melon, and the sweet cucumber. You can identify a pepino by its smooth round or oval shape and its colorful skin, which is light yellow with purple lines throughout. Depending on the type of pepino available, sizes of this fruit vary from small to large.

Therapeutic use: Pepino is a good source of vitamin C, it contains a fair amount of vitamin A and is low in calories.

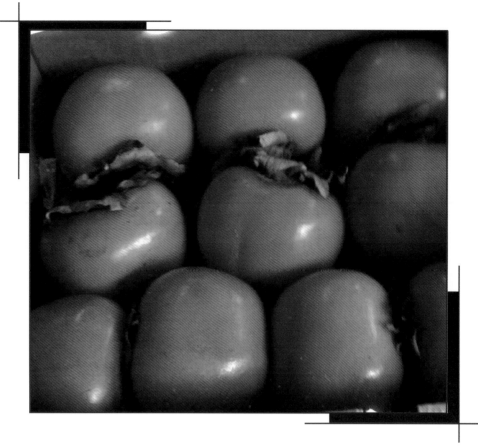

PERSIMMON

Persimmon (Diospyros kaki Linn), known to the ancient Greeks as "the fruit of the gods" is an edible fruit that are generally light yellow-orange to dark red-orange in color, and depending on the species, vary in size from 1.5-9 cm (0.5-4 in) diameter, and may be spherical, acorn-, or pumpkin-shaped. The calyx often remains attached to the fruit after harvesting, but becomes easier to remove as it ripens. They are high in glucose, with a balanced protein profile, and possess various medicinal and chemical uses. While the persimmon fruit is not considered a "common berry" it is in fact a "true berry" by definition.

Commercially, there are generally two types of persimmon fruit: astringent and non-astringent. Fuyu persimmon is by far the most popular and well-known cultivar of persimmons. It is a non-astringent type. Those commercially-available persimmons that shape like an acorn are usually the "Hachiya" cultivar, an astringent persimmon.

Persimmons are eaten fresh or dried, raw or cooked. When eaten fresh the peel is usually cut/peeled off and the fruit is often cut into quarters or eaten whole like an apple. The flesh ranges from firm to mushy and the texture is unique. The flesh is very sweet and when firm possesses an apple-like crunch.

Therapeutic use: Persimmon is low in saturated fat, cholesterol and sodium. It is high in iron and vitamin C.

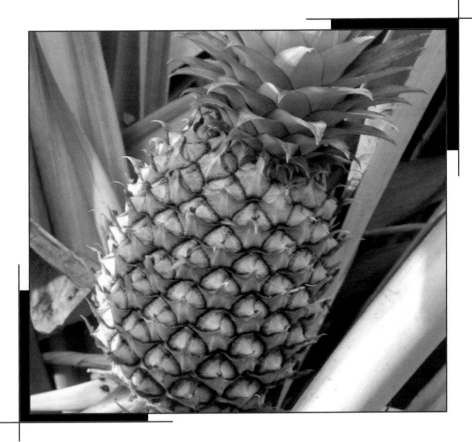

PINEAPPLE

Pineapple (Ananas comosus) is native to the southern part of Brazil and Paraguay. This fruit is eaten fresh or canned and is available as a juice or in juice combinations. It is used in desserts, salads, as a complement to meat dishes and in fruit cocktail.

In Spanish, pineapples are called piña in Spain and most Hispanic American countries or ananá ("ananás", in Argentina). Many languages use the native term ananas. They have varying names in Indian languages: Anaasa in telugu, annachi pazham (Tamil), anarosh (Bengali), and in Malayalam, kaitha chakka. In Malay, pineapples are known as nanas or nenas. A large, sweet pineapple grown especially in Brazil is called abacaxi.

The oval to cylindrical-shaped, compound fruit develops from many small fruits fused together. It is both juicy and fleshy with the stem serving as the fibrous core. Pineapple contains a proteolytic enzyme, bromelain, which breaks down protein. Pineapple juice can thus be used as a marinade and tenderizer for meat.

Southeast Asia dominates world production including Thailand and Philippines.

Therapeutic use: Pineapple is an excellent source of manganese, which is an essential cofactor in a number of enzymes important in energy production and antioxidant defenses. It is also an excellent source of Vitamin C, B1, Copper, dietary fiber and Vitamin B6.

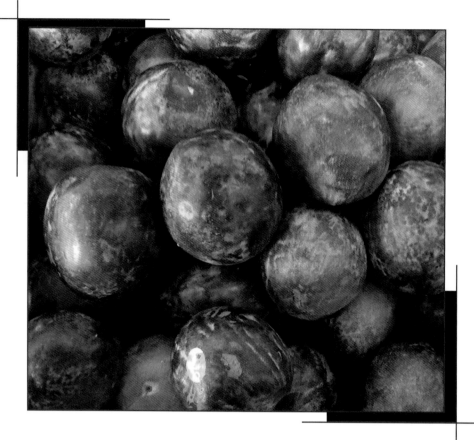

PLUM

Plum or gage (Prunus armeniaca) is a stone fruit tree in the genus Prunus, subgenus Prunus. Plums come in a wide variety of colors and sizes. Some are much firmer-fleshed than others and some have yellow, white, green, orange, purple, pink, black, or red flesh, with equally varying skin color.

Plum fruit is sweet and juicy and it can be eaten fresh or used in jam-making or other recipes. Plum juice can be fermented into plum wine. Dried plums are also called prunes.

Plums are high in sugar, therefore, they have no starch. Consequently, they will not become sweeter after being picked; but their pectic enzymes will dissolve some of the pectin, causing them to soften. This action can be halted with refrigerating. Plums have only moderate amounts of soluble gums and pectins in the flesh, as well as small amounts of cellulose and the noncarbohydrate food fiber lignin in the skin.

Therapeutic use: Plums are a good source of vitamins A and C and potassium, they have very little protein and only a trace of fat, and they do contain more antioxidants than any other fruit.

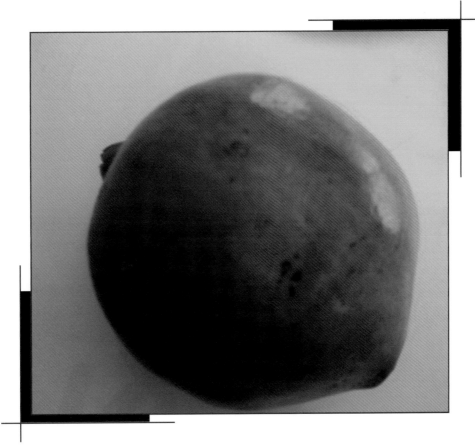

POMEGRANATE

Pomegranate (Punica granatum) is also known as Chinese apple, granada or grenade. It is a popular exotic fruit whose origins are from the Middle East and Asia.

The fruit has a round shape, hard yellow and red colored outer skin, and has an unusual interior flesh that contains many small edible seeds. Pomegranates range in size from three to five inches in length. A semi-sweet pulp that can also be eaten surrounds each of these interior seeds. Additionally, both the seeds and pulp are embedded in a clear membrane. This membrane, although it is also edible, is not very flavorful and is typically not eaten.

Common uses for the pomegranate include eating the fruit raw, using the seeds as dessert toppings and pressing the seeds and pulp to make a juice from them. Pomegranate juice is also used to make salad dressings, wines, jellies and syrups.

Therapeutic use: They provide an excellent source of vitamin C and of fiber. For those counting calories, one pomegranate contains approximately 100 calories.

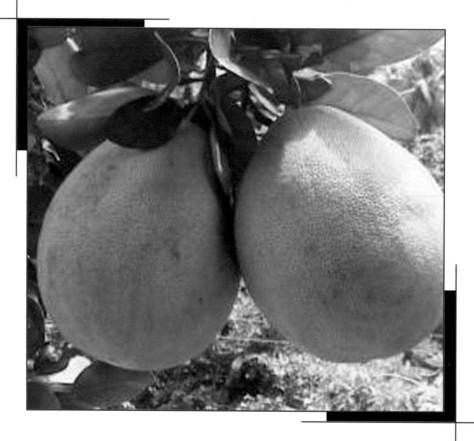

POMELO

Pomelo, (Citrus maxima or Citrus grandis), is a citrus fruit native to South East Asia. It is usually pale green to yellow when ripe, with sweet white (or, more rarely, pink or red) flesh and very thick spongy rind. It is the largest citrus fruit, 15-25 cm in diameter, and usually weighing 1-2 kg. Other names for pomelo include pummelo, pommelo, Chinese grapefruit, jabong, pompelmous, and shaddock. Pomelos are also referred to as chakotara in Pakistan and Afghanistan.

The pomelo tastes like a sweet, mild grapefruit - it has very little or none of the common grapefruit's bitterness, but the membranes of the segments are bitter and usually discarded. The peel is sometimes used to make marmalade, or candied then dipped in chocolate. The peel of the pomelo is also used in Chinese cooking or candied. In general, citrus peel is often used in southern Chinese cuisine for flavoring, especially in sweet soup desserts.

In the Philippines, the fruit is known as the suhâ, or lukban, and is eaten as a dessert or snack. The pommelo, cut into wedges, is dipped in salt before it is eaten, and pommelo is also a flavor for juice drink mixes.

The United States of America is the top producer of pomelo, followed by China, South Africa, Mexico and Israel.

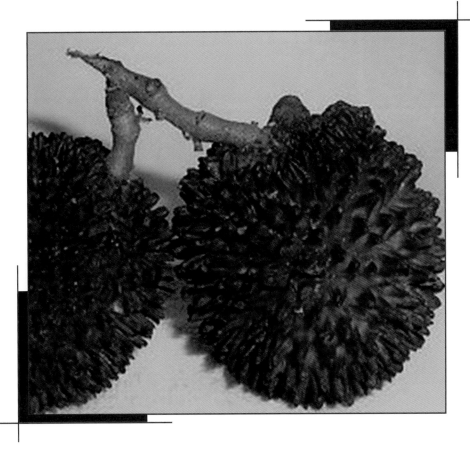

PULASAN

Pulasan (Nephelium mutabile) is a tropical fruit closely allied to the rambutan and sometimes confused with it. It has various common names, including pulasan in English, Spanish and Malay, kapulasan in Malaysia, ngoh-khonsan in Thailand, and bulala in the Philippines.

The fruit is ovoid, 5-7.5 cm long, dark-red, its thick, leathery rind closely set with conical, blunt-tipped tubercles or thick, fleshy, straight spines, to 1 cm long. There may be 1 or 2 small, undeveloped fruits nestled close to the stem. Within is the glistening, white or yellowish-white flesh (aril) to 1 cm thick, more or less clinging to the thin, grayish-brown seedcoat (testa) which separates from the seed. The flavor is generally much sweeter than that of the rambutan. The seed is ovoid, oblong or ellipsoid, light-brown, somewhat flattened on one side, 2-3.5 cm long.

While very similar to rambutan, the fruit lacks the hairy spines. The flesh is very sweet and juicy, and separates easily from the seed, much more easily than the rambutan. In addition, unlike the seed of the rambutan, the seed of the pulasan is readily edible raw, and has a flavor somewhat similar to that of almonds.

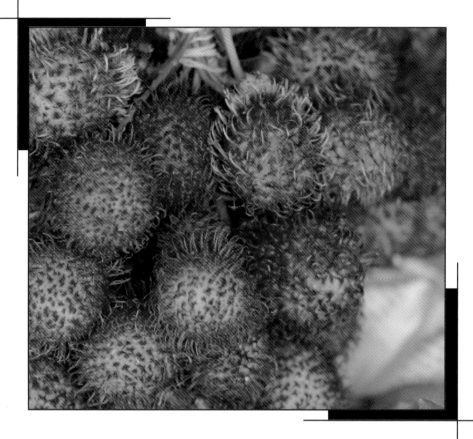

RAMBUTAN

Rambutan (Nephelium lappaceum) is a medium-sized tropical fruit in the family Sapindaceae. It is also known as ramboostan in India; shao tzu in China; chom chom or vai thieu in Vietnam and ser mon or chle sao mon to the Kampucheans.

The fruit is ovoid, or ellipsoid, pinkish-red, bright-or deep-red, orange-red, maroon or dark-purple, yellowish-red, or all yellow or orange-yellow; 1 1/3 to 3 1/8 in (3.4-8 cm) long. Its thin, leathery rind is covered with tubercles from each of which extends a soft, fleshy, red, pinkish, or yellow spine 1/5 to 3/4 in (0.5-2 cm) long, the tips deciduous in some types.

The rambutan is native to Malaysia and commonly cultivated throughout the archipelago and southeast Asia. There are limited plantings in India, a few trees in Surinam, and in the coastal lowlands of Colombia, Ecuador, Honduras, Costa Rica, Trinidad and Cuba. Some fruits are being marketed in Costa Rica. The rambutan was taken to the Philippines from Indonesia in 1912. Further introductions were made in 1920 (from Indonesia) and 1930 (from Malaya), but until the 1950's its distribution was rather limited. Then popular demand brought about systematic efforts to improve the crop and resulted in the establishment of many commercial plantations in the provinces of Batangas, Cavite, Davan, Iloilo, Laguna, Oriental Mindoro and Zamboanga.

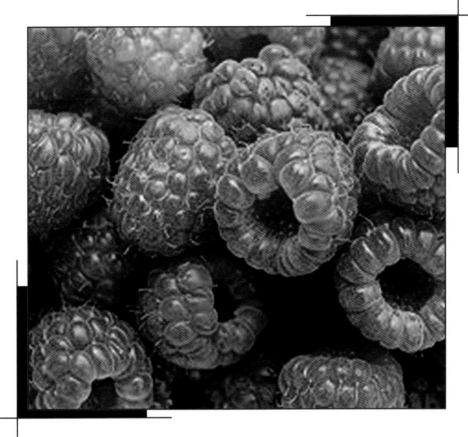

RASPBERRY

Raspberry is the edible fruit of a multitude of plant species in the subgenus Idaeobatus of the genus Rubus; the name also applies to these plants themselves.

Raspberries are red in color, fragrantly sweet with a subtly tart overtone and almost-melt-in-your-mouth texture, raspberries are wonderfully delicious and are usually in limited supply. Most cultivated varieties of raspberries are grown in California from June through October.

A member of the rose family and a bramble fruit like the blackberry, raspberries are delicately structured with a hollow core. Raspberries are known as "aggregate fruits" since they are a compendium of smaller seed-containing fruits, called drupelets, that are arranged around a hollow central cavity.

Therapeutic use: Red raspberry is most often the source of a dietary supplement sold in many health food stores called ellagic acid. This substance found naturally in raspberries belongs to the family of phytonutrients called tannins, and it is viewed as being responsible for a good portion of the antioxidant activity of this (and other) berries.

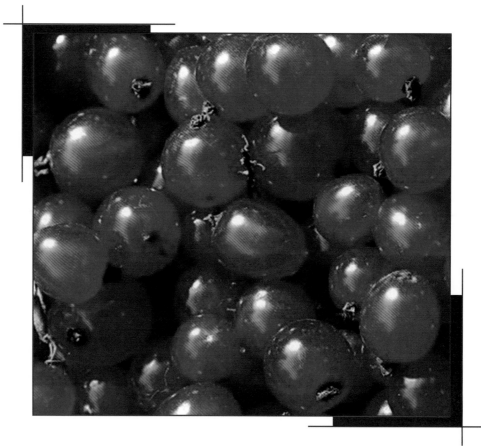

RED CURRANTS

Red Currant (Ribes rubrum) is a member of the genus ribes. It is native to parts of western Europe.

This fruit is slightly more sour than its relative the blackcurrant, and is cultivated mainly for jams and cooked dishes, rather than for eating raw. However, unlike the cranberry, it certainly can be enjoyed in its fresh state and without the addition of sugar.

Therapeutic use: Red currants has high levels of Vitamin C, fruit acids and fiber.

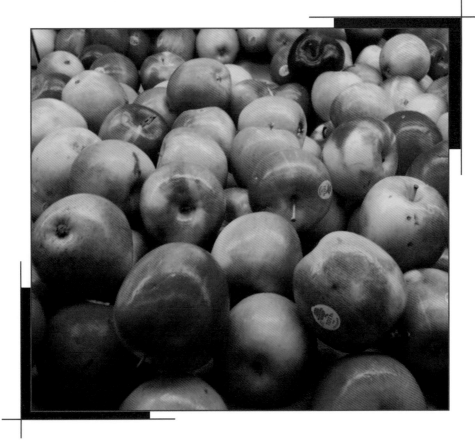

RED DELICIOUS APPLE

Delicious (Red Delicious) Apple, Malus domestica, is an apple cultivar that was recognized in Wellsburg, Iowa in 1880.

It is a medium-sized apple, with a tall conical shape. The dark and intense crimson color makes it the quintessential red apple, and it has a strong shelf appeal. Unfortunately, the visual appeal is not quite matched by the flavor. Red Delicious has a strong sweet flavor, perhaps most reminiscent of slightly overripe melon. It seems like it should be crisp and crunchy, but it is generally too soft.

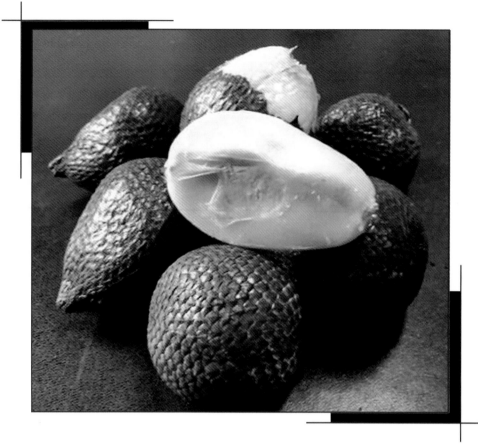

SALAK

Salak (Salacca zalacca) is a species of palm tree native to Indonesia and Malaysia.

The fruit grows in clusters at the base of the palm, and are also known as snake fruit due to the reddish-brown scaly skin. They are about the size and shape of a ripe fig, with a distinct tip.

The pulp is edible. The fruit can be peeled by pinching the tip which should cause the skin to slough off so it can be pulled away. The fruit inside consists of three lobes, each containing a large inedible seed. The lobes resemble, and have the consistency of large peeled garlic cloves. The taste is usually sweet and acidic, but its apple-like texture can vary from very dry and crumbly to moist and crunchy.

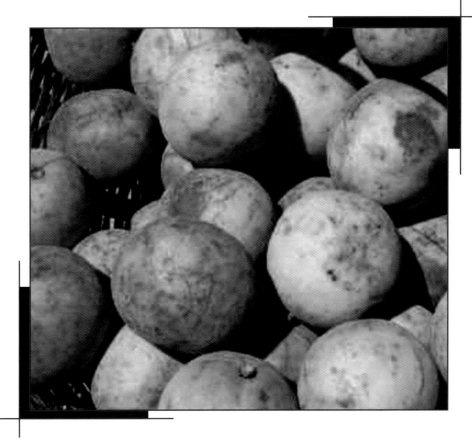

SANTOL

Santol (Sandoricum koetjape) is a tropical fruit grown in southeast Asia.

The tree and its fruit has several common names in many languages, including gratawn in Thai, kompem reach in Khmer, tong in Lao, donka in Sinhalese, and wild mangosteen in English and faux mangoustanier in French.

The Santol is believed native to former Indochina and Peninsular Malaysia, and to have been introduced into India, Borneo, Indonesia, the Moluccas, Mauritius, and the Philippines where it has become naturalized. It is commonly cultivated throughout these regions and the fruits are seasonally abundant in the local markets.

There are two varieties of santol fruit, previously considered two different species, the yellow variety and the red. Both types have a skin that may be a thin peel to a thicker rind. It is edible and contains a milky juice. The pulp may be sweet or sour and contains inedible brown seeds.

Fruit is round and yellow with a very thick skin and segments inside which are very tasty. It is called the "Lolly Fruit" because you have to suck it to get the flavor, as the flesh sticks to the seed. It can be eaten fresh, candied as well prepared into alcoholic beverages.

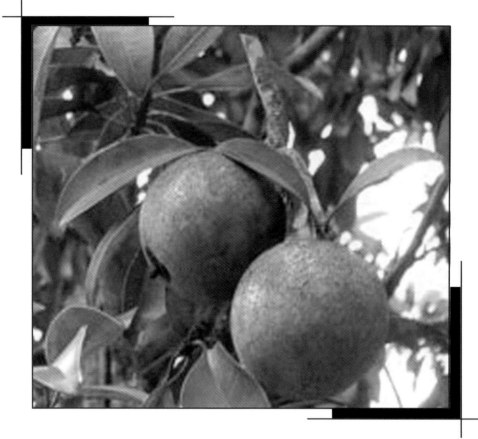

SAPODILLA, CHICO

Sapodilla (Manilkara zapota) is a long-lived, evergreen fruit tree native to Southern Mexico and Central America. It is grown in huge quantities in India, Mexico and was introduced to the Philippines during Spanish colonization.

Sapodilla is known as chikoo (or "chiku,") and sapota in India, sofeda in eastern India and Bangladesh, Sabudheli in Maldives, sawo in Indonesia, hồng xiêm or xa pô chê in Vietnam, lamoot in Thailand and Cambodia, sapodilla in Guyana sapathilla or rata-mi in Sri Lanka, níspero in Colombia, Nicaragua, El Salvador, Dominican Republic and Venezuela, nípero in Cuba, Puerto Rico and Dominican Republic, dilly in The Bahamas, naseberry in the rest of the Caribbean, sapoti in Brazil, and chico sapote in Hawaii, southern California and southern Florida. In Kelantanese Malay, the fruit is called "sawo nilo" which is closer to the original name than the standard Malay "ciku". In Chinese, the name is mistakenly translated by many people roughly as "ginseng fruit", though this is also the name used for the pepino, an unrelated fruit.

The flavor is exceptionally sweet and very tasty, with what can be described as a malty flavor. The unripe fruit is hard to the touch and contains high amounts of saponin, which has astringent properties similar to tannin, drying out the mouth.

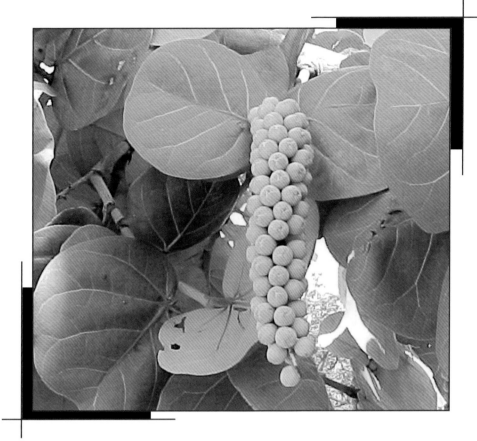

SEA GRAPE

Seagrape (Coccoloba uvifera) is a sprawling bush or small tree that is found near sea beaches throughout tropical America and the Caribbean, including southern Florida, The Bahamas and Bermuda.

Sea grape fruit itself is grape-like although a bit tougher than the ordinary grape and it has one large seed as opposed to several small ones. They remain green and hard for a long time but eventually one by one they change to their mature deep purple color. They hang in bunches, each one with a single seed, and are about the size of regular grapes. When fully mature, they become soft and have a sweet-sour taste making them great for use in jams and jellies. It is possible to make an alcoholic beverage made from the grapes, similar to wine.

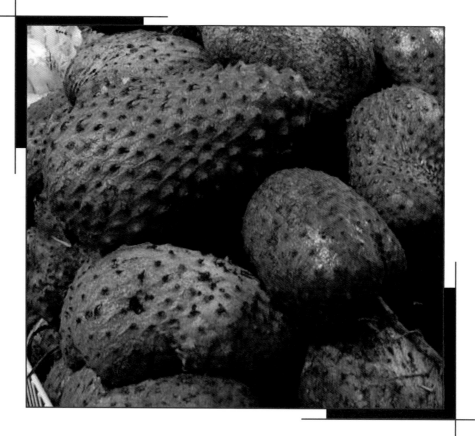

SOURSOP, GUYABANO, GUANABANA

Soursop (Annona muricata), in Spanish it`s guanabana, Portuguese graviola, in Philippines it is known as guyabano.

This fruit is native to the West Indies, today the soursop has spread throughout the humid tropics and is widely grown commercially.

A well-known fruit throughout much of the world, the soursop`s delicious white pulp, with tones of fruit candy and smooth cream is common place in tropical markets, but is rarely found fresh anywhere else. Inside its thin, leathery, green flesh is a large mass of creamy pulp, usually intermixed with 50-100 black seeds.

Therapeutic use: Soursops are high in vitamin B1, B2 and C.

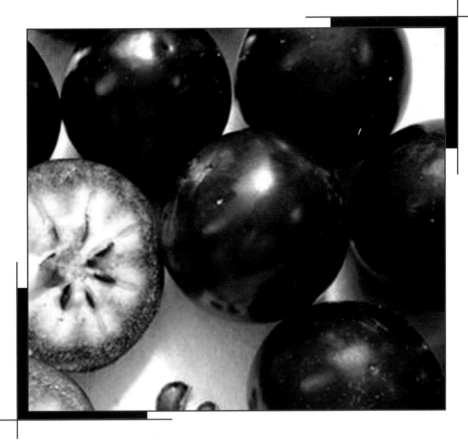

STAR APPLE, CAIMITO

Star Apple (Chrysophyllum cainito), is a tropical fruit native to the lowlands of Central America and West Indies. It has numerous common names including cainito, caimito, milk fruit, aguay, estrella, abiaba and pomme du lait.

The fruit also exist in two colors, dark purple and greenish brown. The purple fruit has a denser skin and texture while the greenish brown fruit has a thin skin and a more liquid pulp.

The fruit has a mild grape-like flavor; it is sweet and is best eaten fresh.

Therapeutic use: It is a good source of vitamin C, known as quercetin.

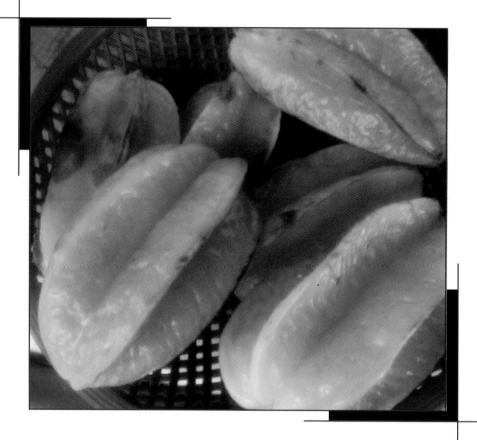

STARFRUIT, CARAMBOLA

Starfruit or carambola (Averrhoa carambola) is a species of tree native to Indonesia, India and Sri Lanka. The tree and its fruit are popular throughout Southeast Asia, Malaysia, the South Pacific and other parts of East Asia. The tree is cultivated also throughout the tropics such as in Trinidad, Guyana, and Brazil, and, in the United States, in south Florida, and Hawaii.

The carambola is closely related to the bilimbi. The fruit in cross section is a five-pointed star, hence its name. Carambolas are best consumed when ripe, when they are yellow with a light shade of green. It will also have brown ridges at the five edges and feel firm. An overripe fruit will be yellow with brown spots.

The fruit is entirely edible, including the slightly waxy skin. It is sweet without being overwhelming and extremely juicy. The taste is difficult to compare, but it has been likened to a mix of papaya, orange and grapefruit all at once.

Therapeutic use: Star fruit is rich in antioxidants and vitamin C, and low in sugar, sodium and acid. Star fruit is a potent source of both primary and secondary polyphenolic antioxidants.

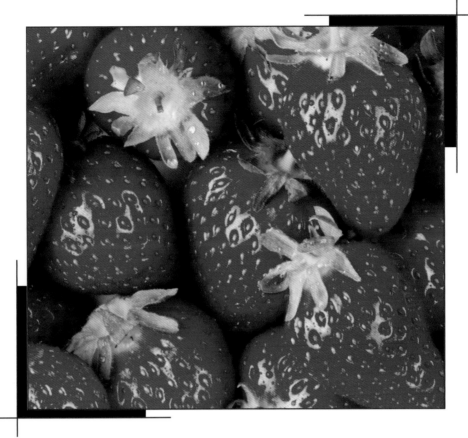

STRAWBERRY

Strawberry, also known as Fragaria, is a genus of flowering plants in the rose family, Rosaceae. There are more than 20 described species and many hybrids and cultivars. The most common strawberries grown commercially are cultivars of the Garden strawberry (Fragaria ×ananassa).

Strawberries have a taste that varies by cultivar, and ranges from quite sweet to rather tart. Strawberries are an important commercial fruit crop, widely grown in all temperate regions of the world.

In addition to being consumed fresh, strawberries can be frozen, made into preserves, as well as dried and used in such things as cereal bars. Strawberries are a popular addition to dairy products, as in strawberry flavored ice cream, milkshakes, smoothies and yogurts. Strawberry pie is also popular.

Therapeutic use: Strawberries are recognized as having more vitamin C than some citrus fruits. They are also high in fiber, folate, potassium and antioxidants, making them a natural means of reducing the chances of heart disease, high blood pressure and certain cancers.

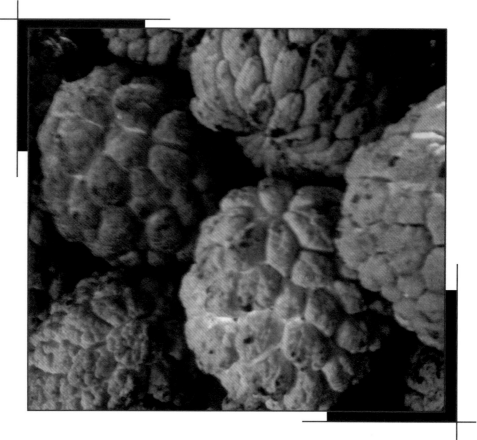

SUGAR APPLE

Sugar-apple (Annona squamosa), also known as sweetsop, is usually round, slightly pine cone-like, 6-10 cm diameter with a scaly or lumpy skin. The fruit flesh is sweet, white to yellow, and resembles and tastes like custard which may be eaten raw.

In English, it is most widely known as sugar-apple or sweetsop. In Taiwan it is called Sakya, aajaa thee in Burma, srikaya in Indonesia, atis in the Philippines, noi-na in Thailand, mang cau ta or na in Vietnam and fruta do conde, pinha or ata in Brazil. In the Middle East region, it is called achta.

It is the most widely cultivated of all species of Annona, being grown widely thoughout the tropics and warmer subtropics such as Indonesia, Thailand, and Taiwan.

Therapeutic use: Sugar-apple fruit is high in calories and is a good source of iron.

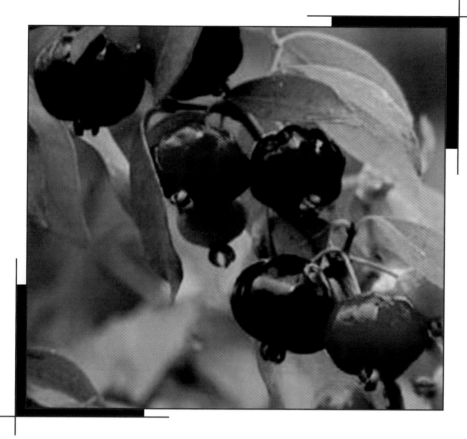

SURINAM CHERRY

Surinam cherry (Eugenia uniflora) is also called pitanga, Brazilian cherry or cayenne cherry.

Surinam cherry itself is a lobed fruit with five to eight ridges. The fruit is dark red or almost black in color and sometimes splits as it ripens. The flesh of the surinam cherry is an orange to red color, very juicy, with two to three small seeds. Surinam cherry tastes acidic with resinous overtones, because the plant produces a great deal of bitter resin.

It is usually eaten fresh, often with sugar or processed into preserves.

Native range extends from Surinam through Uruguay and rarely cultivated outside of the Americas.

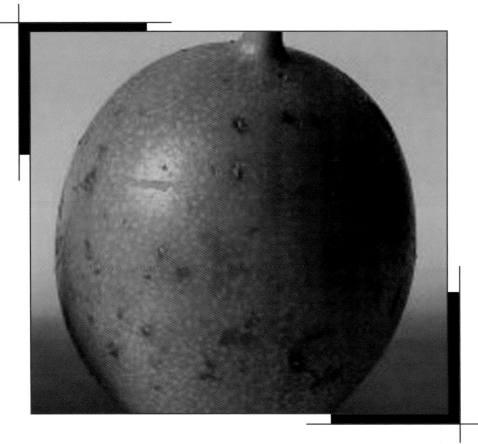

SWEET GRANADILLA

Sweet granadilla (or sometimes called or spelled Grenadia) is one common name for Passiflora ligularis. It is native to the Andes Mountains between Bolivia and Venezuela. It grows as far south as northern Argentina and as far north as Mexico. Outside of its native range it grows in the tropical mountains of Africa and Australia (where they are known as passionfruit).

The fruit is orange to yellow colored with small light markings. It has a round shape with a tip ending in the stem. The fruit is between 6.5 and 8 cm long and between 5.1 and 7 cm in diameter. The outer shell is hard and slippery, and has soft padding on the interior to protect the seeds. The seeds, which are hard and black, are surrounded by a gelatinous sphere of transparent pulp. The pulp is the edible part of the fruit and has a soft sweet taste.

The main producers are Peru, Venezuela, Colombia, Ecuador, Brazil, South Africa, and Kenya. The main importers are the United States, Canada, Belgium, Holland, Switzerland, and Spain.

Therapeutic use: It is very aromatic and contains Vitamins A, C, and K, Phosphorus, Iron, and Calcium.

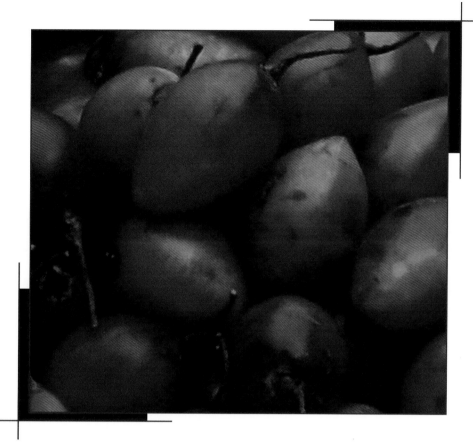

TAMARILLO

Tamarillo, tree tomato, or tomate de árbol is the edible fruit of Solanum betaceum, a species of small tree or shrub in the flowering plant family Solanaceae. It is egg-shaped, with a thin deep red or yellow skin and a soft flesh (when ripe), with dark-colored seeds occupying about one third of the interior.

The fruit can be between 2 and 8 cm in length. They are held on the tree in clusters as are many other clustered fruit, such as cherries.

The tamarillo is native to the Andes of Peru, Chile, Ecuador and Bolivia. It is cultivated in Argentina, Australia, Brazil, Colombia, Indonesia (where it is known as "terong Belanda" or "Dutch eggplant"), Kenya, Portugal, the United States and Venezuela. It is grown as a commercial crop for international export in New Zealand and Portugal.

The fruit is eaten by scooping the flesh from a halved fruit, but in New Zealand children palpate the ripe fruit until it is soft then bite off the stem end and squeeze the flesh directly into their mouths. The flesh of the tamarillo is tangy and mildly sweet, and may be compared to kiwifruit, tomato, or passion fruit. The skin and the flesh near it have an unpleasant bitter taste, and usually aren't eaten raw.

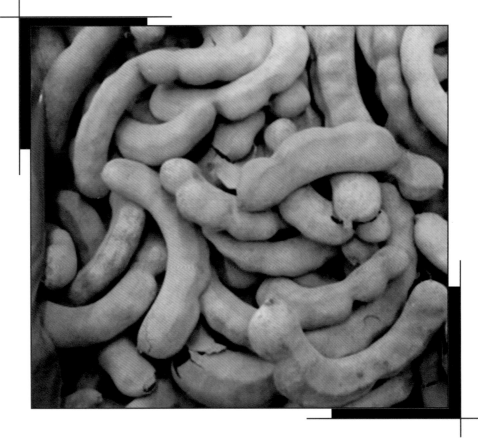

TAMARIND

Tamarind (Tamarindus indica) is a tropical fruit, native to Africa, including Sudan and parts of the Madagascar dry deciduous forests. Alternative names include Indian date, translation of Arabic tamr hindī. In Indonesia it is called asem (or asam) Jawa (means Javanese asam) in Indonesian. In Malaysia it is called asam in Malay. In the Philippines it is called sampaloc in Tagalog and sambag in Cebuano. In Oriya it is called tentuli. In Bengali it is known as tentul. In Hindi and in Urdu it is called imli. in Gujarati it is called amli. In Marathi and Konkani it is called chinch. In Bangla, the term is tētul. In Sinhala the name is siyambala, in Telugu it is called chintachettu (tree) and chintapandu (fruit extract) and in Tamil and Malayalam it is puli. In Kannada it is called hunase. In Malagasy it is called voamadilo. The Vietnamese term is me. In Colombia, Mexico, Puerto Rico and Venezuela it is called tamarindo. In the US Virgin Islands, tamarind is sometimes called tamon, in Thailand it is called ma-kham. In Taiwan it is called loan-tz. In Myanmar it is called magee-thee.

The fruit pulp is edible and popular. The hard green pulp of a young fruit is very sour and acidic, so much it cannot be consumed directly, but is often used as a component of savory dishes. The ripened fruit is edible, as it becomes less sour and somewhat sweeter, but still very acidic. It is used in desserts as a jam, blended into juices or sweetened drinks, or as a snack.

Therapeutic use: It is also consumed as a natural laxative.

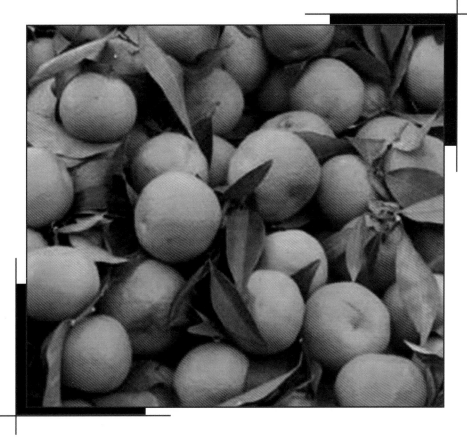

TANGERINE

Tangerine (Citrus × tangerina) is an orange-colored citrus fruit. It is a variety of the Mandarin orange (Citrus reticulata). Tangerine fruit is flattened in shape, 2 to 4 inches in diameter, and orange-red in color. The rind is thin and leathery and peels from the fruit easily. The taste is often less sour, or tart, than that of an orange.

Tangerines are most commonly peeled and eaten out of hand. The fresh fruit is also used in salads, desserts and main dishes. Fresh tangerine juice and frozen juice concentrate are commonly available in the United States.

Therapeutic use: Tangerines are a good source of vitamin C, folate and beta-carotene. They also contain some potassium, magnesium and vitamins B1, B2 & B3. Tangerine oil, like all citrus oils, has limonene as its major constituent, but also alpha-pinene, myrcene, gamma-terpinene, citronellal, linalool, neral, neryl acetate, geranyl acetate, geraniol, thymol, and carvone.

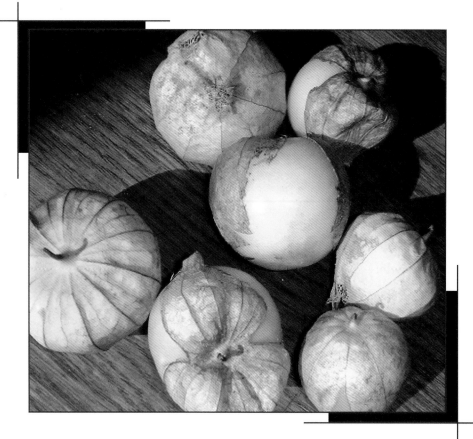

TOMATILLOS

Tomatillo (Physalis philadelphica), is a fruit related to tomatoes, which is small, spherical and green or green-purple. Tomatillos, referred to as green tomato in Mexico, are a staple in Mexican cuisine. Tomatillos are grown throughout the Western Hemispere. They should not be confused with green unripe tomatoes (Tomatoes are of the same family but of different genus).

Tomatillo is also known as the husk tomato, jamberry, husk cherry, Mexican tomato, or ground cherry.

The fruit is surrounded by a paper-like husk formed from the calyx. As the fruit matures, it fills the husk and can split it open by harvest. The husk turns brown, and the fruit can be any of a number of colors when ripe, including yellow, red, green or even purple.

Tomatillos are the key ingredient in fresh and cooked Latin American green sauces.

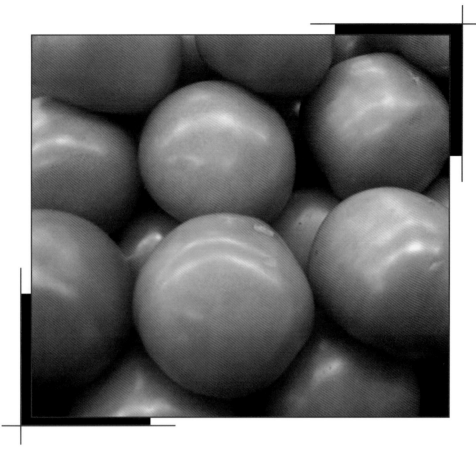

TOMATO

Tomato is a delicious, nutritious fruit, more widely known as a vegetable. Botanically, a tomato (Solanum lycopersicum) is the ovary of a flowering plant, therefore it is a fruit, or, more specifically, a berry. However, since it's not as sweet as other fruits and is most often served in salads or as a main dish - most people refer to it as a vegetable.

More than 125 tons of tomatoes are produced in the world today with China being the largest producer, followed by the United States and Turkey.

Therapeutic use: Tomatoes are high in Vitamin A and C and are naturally low in calories. They are also an excellent source of lycopene, which is the pigment that makes tomatoes red and has been linked to the prevention of many types of cancer. Lycopene is an antioxidant which fights free radicals that can interfere with normal cell growth and activity. These free radicals are what can potentially lead to cancer, heart disease and premature aging. The best sources of lycopene are found in processed tomato products, such as ketchup and tomato products.

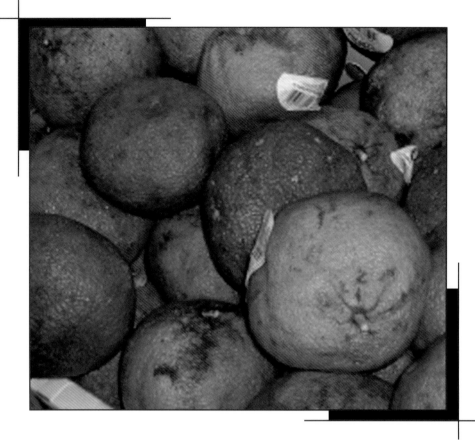

UGLI FRUIT

Ugli fruit is a Jamaican tangelo, a citrus fruit created by hybridizing a grapefruit (or pomelo according to some sources) and a tangerine. Its species is Citrus reticulata x Citrus paradisi.

It was discovered growing wild in Jamaica where it is mainly grown today. Its name derives from the unsightly appearance of its rough, wrinkled, greenish-yellow skin, wrapped loosely around the orange pulpy citrus inside. The light green surface blemishes turn orange when the fruit is at its peak ripeness. An ugli fruit is usually slightly larger than a grapefruit (but this varies) and has fewer seeds. The flesh is very juicy and tends towards the sweet side of the tangerine rather than the bitter side of its grapefruit lineage, with a fragrant skin. The taste is often described as more sour than an orange and less bitter than a tangerine, however, and is more commonly guessed to be a lemon-tangerine hybrid.

The fruit is also described as an exotic tangelo.

Ugli are easily peeled and may be eaten like a tangerine, or cut in half and eaten like a grapefruit. The pegs and juice may be used to make many sumptuous sweet and savory recipes.

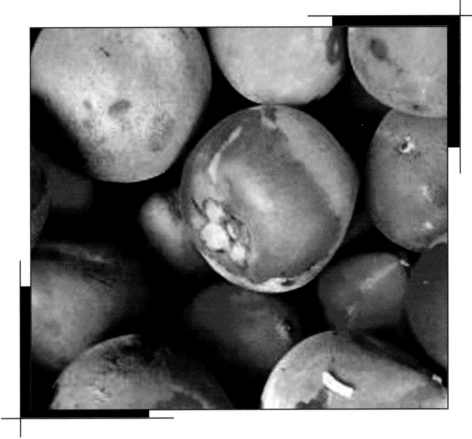

VELVET APPLE, MABOLO

Velvet Apple (Diospyros blancoi), also called mabolo, is a very beautiful dark purple colored fruit with velvet-like skin. Fruit is about the size of an apple, with mildly sweet flavored, somewhat mealy flesh. Fruits are highly esteemed in some areas, but rarely known in most parts of the world.

It is usually eaten fresh out of hand or used in salads and desserts.

The mabolo is indigenous to the low and medium altitude forests of the Philippine Islands from the island of Luzon to the southernmost of the Sulu Islands, and is commonly cultivated for its fruit and even more as a shade tree for roadsides. The tree was introduced into Java and Malaya, and, in 1881, into Calcutta and the Botanical Garden in Singapore, though it existed in Singapore before that date.

Therapeutic use: The fruit is considered a fairly good source of iron and calcium and a good source of vitamin B.

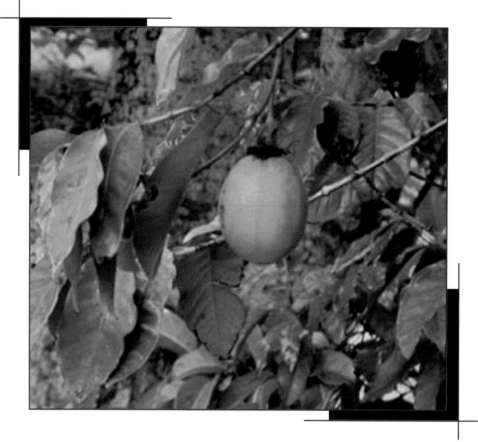

WATER LEMON

Water Lemon (Passiflora laurifolia), also called bell apple, yellow granadilla or golden apple, is a medium sized, ovaloid fruit, usually with a deep orange skin and white-yellow, extremely juicy pulp. The water lemon has an excellent perfumy-mild taste, without the tartness of the common passion fruit. A not widely known, and very underrated passion fruit.

It is eaten fresh or used in drinks. Native to tropical America. It is an invasive plant in tropical regions and has spread to many other parts of the world. Only occasionally cultivated, but fruits are usually available in markets wherever the vine grows wild.

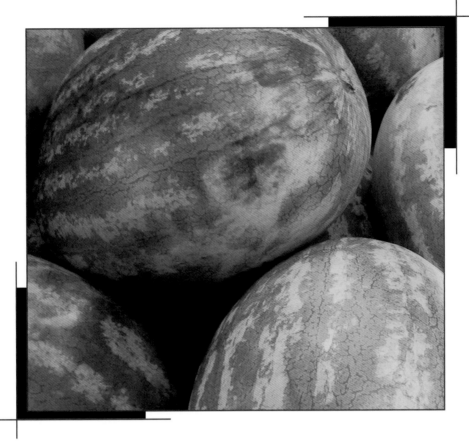

WATERMELON

Watermelon (Citrullus lanatus) is originally from southern Africa and one of the most common types of melon. The watermelon fruit, loosely considered a type of melon (although not in the genus Cucumis), has a smooth exterior rind (green, yellow, and sometimes white) and a juicy, sweet, usually red, but sometimes orange, yellow, or pink interior flesh.

Fresh watermelon may be eaten in a variety of ways and is also often used to flavor summer drinks and smoothies.

There are more than twelve hundred varieties of watermelon ranging in size from less than a pound, to more than two hundred pounds with flesh that is red, orange, yellow, or white.

Therapeutic use: Watermelon contains about six percent sugar by weight, the rest being mostly water. As with many other fruits, it is a source of vitamin C. It is not a significant source of other vitamins and minerals unless one eats several kilograms per day.

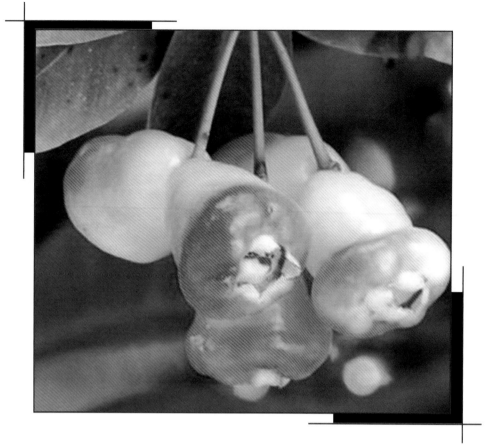

WAX APPLE, WAX JAMBU, MACOPA

Wax apple (Syzygium samarangense) is also called Java apple, love apple, Chompu (in Thai), bellfruit (in Taiwan), jambu air (in Indonesia), water apple, mountain apple, jambu air (water guava) in Malay, wax jambu, rose apple, bell fruit, makopa, tambis (in Philippines), and chambekka in Malayalam and jumbu (in Sri lanka).

It is a pear shaped fruit with waxy skin and crispy flesh similar to the malay apple. Fruit is often juicy, with a subtle sweet taste somewhat resembling a common apple. Superior varieties are of excellent quality.

Almost always eaten fresh. Bland varieties are often eaten with sugar sprinkled over the flesh.

Native to Malaysia, Philippines and some islands of Indonesia. Often cultivated in southeast Asia, but rarely grown elsewhere. Fruits are occasionally imported to Canada and Europe.

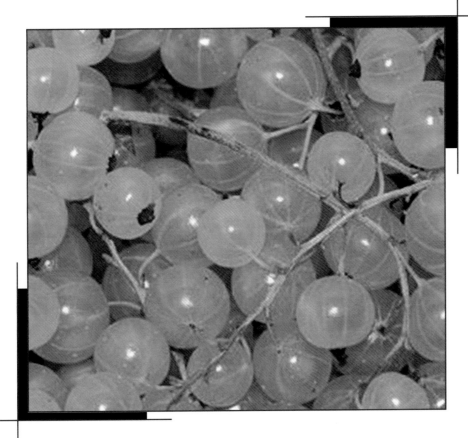

WHITE CURRANT

White Currant (whitecurrant) is also a common cultivar of red currant. It is sometimes called yellow currant and is a member of the genus Ribes.

White currant berries are a bit smaller and sweeter than red currants. Although white currants seem to be used less in cooking than their red counterparts, and more for eating raw, white currant jellies, wines and syrups are not unheard of. They are sometimes used to make "pink" jams and jellies (a mixture of white and red). The white currant is actually an albino cultivar of the redcurrant, but is marketed as a different fruit.

Therapeutic use: They are a good source of vitamins B1 and C, and are rich in iron, copper and manganese. Dried currants are highly alkalinizing. Pink currants are a hybrid of red and white.

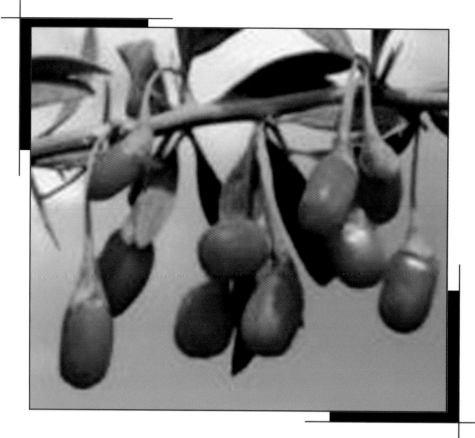

WOLFBERRY

Wolfberry, commercially called goji berry, is the common name for the fruit of two very closely related species: Lycium barbarum and L. chinense, two species of boxthorn in the family Solanaceae. It is native to southeastern Europe and Asia.

It is also known as Chinese wolfberry, goji berry, mede berry, barbary matrimony vine, bocksdorn, Duke of Argyll's tea tree, Murali (in India), red medlar or matrimony vine.

The fruit is a bright orange-red, ellipsoid berry 1-2 cm long. The number of seeds in each berry varies widely based on cultivar and fruit size, containing anywhere between 10-60 tiny yellow seeds that are compressed with a curved embryo.

Wolfberries are almost never found in their fresh form outside of their production regions, and are usually sold in open boxes and small packages in dried form. As a food, dried wolfberries are traditionally cooked before consumption.

Therapeutic use: Wolfberry fruits have been used since ancient times in China as general tonic, to protect the liver, to improve vision, to strengthen weak legs and to promote longevity.

FRUITS OF THE WORLD
Therapeutic Uses
Health, Prevention, Medicines

Dr.Kumar Pati Describes:

FRUITS ARE FROM HEAVEN
Their Health Benefits

- Provides the source of enzyme
- Good nutrients for digestion
- Powerful antioxidants
- Contains colorful pigmentation
- Increases Energy
- Promotes immune system
- Powerful Anti-Ageing Properties
- Promotes longevity
- The best source of Vitamin C
- Reduces sleeping Problem
- Promotes eye health (night blindness)
- Promotes Prostate health
- Helps liver and Spleen disorder
- Improves Circulation
- Strengthens immune System
- Acts as a good immunomodulator
- Eases headache and dizziness
- Promotes skin health
- Anti-asthmatic
- Stabilizes blood pressures
- Promotes cardio vascular health
- Prevents strokes
- Reduces plasma lipids
- Best source of monosaturated fats
- Increases metabolic rates
- Contains anti-inflammatory effects
- A good source of daily nutritional regimen